A Guide to
Practice Based

A GUIDE TO PRACTICE BASED COMMISSIONING

by Steve Williams AFA FIAB MIHM

Published in the UK by
Magister Consulting Ltd
The Old Rectory
St. Mary's Road
Stone
Dartford
Kent DA9 9AS

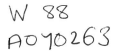
Copyright © 2006 Magister Consulting Ltd
Printed in the UK by Nuffield Press Ltd, Abingdon, Oxon.

ISBN 1 873839 68 5

About the author

Steve Williams (AFA, FIAB, MIHM) is a qualified accountant and a member of the Institute of Healthcare Management who has worked within the NHS for over 20 years, and has previously written books on Fundholding and on Making Best Practice Better. He currently provides practice management expertise to many medical practices and also acts as an accountant for GPs. He has worked with PMS Contracts and, more recently, has been assisting doctors to assess the implications of the new GMS Contract.

Steve Williams has also been an associate tutor for the Institute of Health Policy Studies at the University of Southampton and has written many articles and training modules on GP practice.

Acknowledgements

Thank you to my staff, who have supported me and my work within Primary Care for many years, and to all the many clients I have worked with throughout many periods of dynamic change.

Foreword

By the time this book is published, there will already be a number of published articles or papers relating to practice based commissioning. Many will concentrate on the role of the Primary Care Trust (PCT), Strategic Health Authority (SHA) or Hospital Trust. Some will focus on primary care, but will mainly tackle the core framework of how the system will potentially operate.

This book will look at how practice based commissioning will impact on an already busy general practice and, with this in mind, its purpose is to assist the general practice in adopting its own approach to ensure it is best ready to meet the demands of this new initiative. The core competency framework for managers covers many areas and, where appropriate, cross-referencing within the book will assist in delivering these competencies.

The book has also been written for General Practitioners (GPs) in order that they can quickly evaluate the amount of work needed to implement the initiative, and be better able to understand the increasing demands being placed on management. It will allow them to be supportive of the process and ensure that there is adequate reward for the amount of effort required to achieve the necessary changes.

Primary care is clearly being asked to do more and more; at a time when we have the new contract, Working in Partnership Programme, Primary Care Collaboratives, Medicines Management, Choose and Book, Access Targets and Patient Choice, to name but a few, it is imperative that effectiveness is maintained by the use of knowledge management. Knowledge Management is formulated on the concept that a practice's most valuable resource is the knowledge of its staff. The effectiveness of the practice will be measured, in part, on how efficiently its staff can create or develop new knowledge, share that knowledge around the practice and use that knowledge to best effect.

Practice based commissioning is not currently governed by strict guidelines and therefore, as PCTs develop their own approach as to how they will work in their own specific locality, this knowledge will become available and can then be shared. Consider this book as being the thoughts of your own Effective Manager, who has researched the knowledge to date concerning practice based commissioning, who has developed this knowledge, and is now sharing that knowledge with you. At the end of each chapter, reference has been made to what the Effective Manager should be considering.

Steve Williams AFA FIAB MIHM

September 2005

Contents

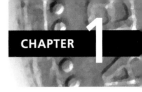
Introduction - a brief history

The white paper of 1998 identified that practice based commissioning would eventually be rolled out to all practices for a full range of services. From April 2005 practices had the opportunity to apply for indicative commissioning budgets. In reality many PCTs were not ready to engage in discussions with practices expressing an interest. That is not true in all areas, because good work has been done in establishing local commissioning models in many parts of the country. However, this was the first time that the practice itself had the opportunity to express a direct interest in taking part. Does this differ from fundholding? The answer is that in part it is exactly what fundholding was about, i.e. a devolved budget and a measurement of activity against cost. However, the new concept of commissioning is looking at only devolving an indicative budget, and instead of merely being a way of reducing costs and potentially waiting times, it will look at a variety of new issues such as quality and variety.

The biggest problem facing anyone involved in commissioning is recognising the top down approach to funding and the bottom up approach of demand. The divergence of these two approaches means that there is still the potential for cost and service inequalities to develop.

By devolving the financial budgets to primary care, albeit indicative, weight will be added to the importance of patient choice. Practices will need to meet this demand by securing a wider range of services into their commissioning model; services more responsive to the direct needs of their patients. Additionally, the implementation of choose and book and, by 2008, the opportunity for patients to choose elective procedures, means that the practice must be planning now how it is going to deal with these changes. One of the obvious opportunities is the development of practice based services, meaning that primary care itself can offer an alternative or greater choice to patients. How will it be funded? Well, the idea is that there will be a system of payment by results or in other words funding will follow the patient. Also expected to benefit will be those patients who need packages of care, such as the terminally ill or those with long-term chronic conditions.

Key aims

The practice based commissioning model should have the following key aims:

- Increase the range and variety of services offered

- Increase the number of service providers and add greater choice

- Offer more convenient locations to patients

- Create a more efficient use of total NHS services and resources

- Involve primary care clinical staff in direct commissioning decisions.

Many of the major stakeholders within the NHS are already endorsing a variety of different commissioning models with the key factor being that the process involves those clinicians working within primary care. Years ago GPs were described as the gatekeepers and that has not really changed; it is still primary care that will act as the main instigator of the utilisation of NHS services over the longer term. Many of the components needed to make practice based commissioning work are already in place or have been tried and tested to a fuller or lesser degree over the last few years. It is likely that PCTs will drive forward programmes to involve all practices in commissioning, whether as groups or as individuals.

What can the practice expect? It is envisaged that a practice that engages in the commissioning of services will be able to inform the budget setting process and assist in the risk management of services. The practice will be able to recoup reasonable management costs for administering the process and be able to use any efficiency gains created.

Practice based commissioning is a process for assessing the needs locally for patients and ensuring that appropriate budget is allocated to those clinicians who have identified those services. The PCT will continue to act as the custodian of the actual funds and be responsible for the administrative support role necessary to allow commissioning to work effectively.

Good practice management is imperative in ensuring that this initiative works effectively. The core competency framework defines certain levels of ability for the different levels of management within the practice. The following chapters will make reference to these competencies, where they will be applicable to practice based commissioning.

The Institute of Healthcare Managers (IHM) is already looking at a range of competencies for practice management. It envisages the role of the competent manager and at a higher level, the excellent manager. Ultimately, the IHM will be looking for chartered status. This progression of professionalism means that the practice manager at the heart of all the new initiatives being unveiled at general practice level must be able to embrace an extensive range of skills and abilities. This book will hopefully allow the already busy manager to acquire an all round knowledge of the principles of practice based commissioning, and at the end of each chapter, reference will be made to what an effective manager should be considering.

The Effective Manager

1. Gain an understanding of the earlier models of commissioning. During fundholding, both software and statutory instruments were developed that allowed a purchaser/ provider regime to be created. The models that developed from these early days can still be applied today.

2. Document your own practice's current referral pattern and, if it is still available, compare this to referral patterns that were documented during the times of fundholding or more latterly locality commissioning.

3. Consider how the practice commissioned services during this time, particularly if alternative providers were used or if in-house services were utilised. If a practice commissioned services one way in the past, are they relevant now? If they are, then does the practice want to explore this avenue again? If so, it may be able to tap into the wealth of experience gained previously.

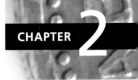

Which services can be commissioned?

How long is a piece of string? Before a practice can decide which services to commission, it must consider a number of other local factors. Firstly, the practice must be clear about why it wishes to undertake the commissioning process. This should be defined by the amount of effort needed to generate any expected outcomes. The practice will need to look at its own existing referral patterns and patient needs. In some areas the needs will already be sufficient to meet local commissioning guidelines in respect of levels of service, but in others there will not be the capacity to allow services to be commissioned. The latter can be resolved by the use of collaborative commissioning, where more than one practice enters into a joint agreement, normally in discussion with, and support of, the Primary Care Trust.

The range of services commissioned in the first year may reflect the future level or range of services commissioned. The whole process will be reactive to local needs and patient demand. Of course, it will not be as simple as stating the preferred commissioning levels; the proposed level of service will need to be agreed with the Primary Care Trust who in turn will need to reach agreement with their Professional Executive Committee (PEC). This is to ensure that there is equality and transparency across the whole Trust practice population.

The PCT will not place unnecessary restrictions upon the range of services to be commissioned, but they will be responsible for ensuring that any services commissioned are viable and will consider the needs arising as a result of changing commissioning patterns. They will also need to plan for any unexpected requirements and be aware of how these may impact the delivery of services as a whole.

Practices, particularly those that took part in fundholding, will be aware of the process of commissioning and decisions can be made now whether or not to apply for a full range of services or just to select a limited range. What should be noted is that although practices may embark on this process at any time from 1st April 2005, a true full range of services, which would include all outpatient and emergency admissions, will not be available during 2005 and 2006.

What can the indicative budget actually mean?

Whatever the budget held, each practice is entitled to receive information about their use of available health services. All practices currently receive detailed information about their prescribing, but not all PCTs have developed a system to inform practices about their use of other services. Information is available about community services, such as attached staff (District Nurses, etc.) but little information is available about other services.

The future of any practice based commissioning model will be dependant on a measurable set of outcomes. The healthcare commission will almost certainly insist that this information forms the basis of any good model.

The local delivery plan

In order to achieve an effective plan, it will be important to consider many factors. Firstly, will practices work independently or collectively, and which is more effective? Already those that were involved in fundholding commissioning will recognise the potential models emerging: a single practice; a consortium of two or three practices; a larger group; locality based commissioning; special interest groups; and so on. It should be remembered that although the concepts are not new, the administration of this particular version of the scheme is new and untested. The key difference this time is that there will be genuine opportunities for local innovation and this will cause a wide range of interpretation of how commissioning will develop in each PCT area.

One of the key factors relating to practice based commissioning is whether the practice itself is ready to accept a budget. Given that most practices are still coming to terms with the new contract, access targets, primary care collaborative initiatives, quality outcomes framework, choose and book, patient choice and understanding the core competency framework, it is not known at what point the practice will feel comfortable about accepting a budget. Although there is provision to charge reasonable management costs against future savings, many PCTs are already top-slicing or imposing a charge against any savings before these reasonable costs are achieved. This may actually act as a deterrent to many practices taking up early participation in the scheme.

The real difference between this and previous commissioning models is that it is designed to incorporate so many facets of the NHS as part of the commissioning process. The practice will be involved, the providers will be involved (both NHS and private), patients, community groups, other clinicians (not just GPs), the PCT, Strategic Health Authority and the Healthcare Commission. This is not withstanding those professional organisations that form part of the Working in Partnership Programme *(see Appendix K)*, who will still want to add their viewpoint to the development of the scheme.

Have things really changed?

The whole concept of holding a budget means some inequalities will exist at the start of the scheme, as with most new innovations of this type. If a practice is historically a high referrer it will in essence be rewarded in year one, simply by being funded on an historical basis. This is to the detriment of the low referrer, who will receive a smaller allocation. This is why PCTs already prefer to group practices together to try and balance out the numbers of referrals between practices. Over time and using weighted capitation (pound per patient), it is envisaged that the budgets will be equalised accordingly. However, let us not forget that the underpinning resources available for this initiative are already below what is needed.

Consequently, it will be important to understand the actual patient needs attached to a referral pattern. If there is a genuine need, then the practice should not be penalised for delivering patient care that forms part of the local delivery plan. However, it is only the practice that truly knows its own needs and it now has the task of ensuring that these needs are identified in the local delivery plan (LDP). If these needs are not recognised and the practice starts to overspend, it could lead to the practice being blamed for overspending and as a result, it could lose its commissioning status.

What might a small practice expect?

A practice of say list size 4000 will expect in year one to receive a limited budget. In year two it might expect to receive an extended budget and consider joining and working with two other practices. In year three it will hold a total budget. In year one the practice will be funded on an historic basis. In year two this historic budget will be adjusted by local factors identified in the merger with the other two practices. In year three the budget will be funded using weighted capitation.

The above is just a hypothetical example of what will happen, but it is illustrative of how commissioning models will develop. As a result of practice based commissioning and the new contract, there are PCTs that have actively been encouraging smaller practices to form new Personal Medical Services (PMS) or General Medical Services (GMS) agreements to allow formal mergers to take place.

The practice should not expect to have to elect for any particular model at any given time. They should be aware of their rights and allow their PCT to advise them of what is available locally. Being honest, there is an underlying theme to joint commissioning and it is brought about by the economies of scale. Pooling resources means that there can be a sharing of duties. For example, each practice may not need to have a commissioning lead; there may only need to be one per commissioning group. Attached clinical staff, such as specialist nurses, can be shared accordingly. Management and administration costs can be pooled.

The following describes the competencies already expected from the practice in certain areas:

Clinical services

The Administrator will ensure that current data is available to inform decisions about service provision and may also be able to assist in identifying areas of need. This might be taken from local knowledge of certain regular clinics, such as well woman clinics, baby clinics or minor surgery.

The Manager will review the current practice service provision and will be in a position to recommend changes to the way services are offered. For example, based on their knowledge of influenza vaccination uptake, they might determine how vaccines will be administered by organising clinics at pre-determined times for maximum efficiency, or extending their services to patients of other practices.

The Strategist will take overall responsibility for the service requirements and will comment upon new services or changes to existing provision. They will review demand on certain services and consider the amount of services provided, when and where they are provided, and who provides them. There can be greater flexibility now within practice, and nurses can take on more tasks themselves, supported by healthcare assistants. This can then free time for the GP or allow time to undertake other work.

The Effective Manager

1. The speed at which services can be commissioned will be determined locally. However, as a practice you should draw up a schedule of services and identify the level of usage against each area. As more services become incorporated into the commissioning strategy, you will be ready to assume responsibility for inclusion in the indicative budget.

2. Draw up your own indicative budget by comparing cost against activity. As time goes on more information will become available in the form of published tariffs. When you are awarded your indicative budget, compare your model with what is offered and therefore understand how local cost pressures are going to influence how you effectively manage your own budget.

3. As soon as possible obtain an up-to-date version of the local delivery plan. Understanding what the PCT strategy is will help shape your own intentions. It may also highlight areas where your own practice does not conform to the local average patient needs. Sometimes demographics can cause there to be isolated pockets of health needs. If your practice falls into one of these categories, then practice based commissioning should, over a period of time, help to reshape services to meet these previously unmet needs.

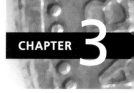

CHAPTER 3

Producing your business plan and being accountable

You may well ask why the need for a business plan? Well, as with most things in the NHS, we need to be able to demonstrate appropriate spending of public money, including value for money and quality of services. So, as with most initiatives, the practice will be expected to have sound management and organisational controls in place. This should not be a major problem for practices. PMS practices already need to produce and report on annual PMS plans. The Quality and Outcomes Framework (QOF) has already been successful in demonstrating the organisational abilities of general practice. The only real difference with this plan is that it needs to be sympathetic to the needs of both the PCT requirements (NHS) and local health needs (patient).

Understand the commissioning cycle

To be able to produce an effective plan, it is necessary to understand the process. Under the core competency framework, reference has been made to PDSA (Plan, Do, Study, Act – *see Appendix C*) cycles. The idea behind this concept is that you plan and then evaluate, producing new PDSA cycles as a result. The initial planning cycle for commissioning includes the following components:

1. Identify health needs and ensure patient involvement

2. Consider national targets

3. Consider the local delivery plan

4. Identify capacity – look at historic usage and planned future usage

5. Consider service redesign, development and providers

6. Enter into Service Level Agreements

7. Monitor performance

8. Identify health needs, i.e. start the process again for next year.

The basic components

Practice based commissioning is to be governed by a financial system called 'payment by results'. This system is designed to pay for activity when it is actually undertaken at a national tariff price. For this to work, budgets need to be devolved to local PCT level and then to practices as an indicative budget. PCTs will receive funding allocations spanning a period of three years, allowing greater flexibility for planning local services.

Investment has been promised with the caveat that it should be spent wisely and must represent excellent value for money. Provider status has been opened up to create a wider choice of service delivery and finally there is patient choice. Patient choice will be key to the process, because the introduction of choose and book means that patients will now be allowed to choose from at least four or five hospitals for elective procedures.

The QOF aspect of the new contract and its focus on chronic illnesses mean that the practice is already introducing effective local personal patient care. This work, when evaluated, will be seen to have an impact on referral patterns within general practice. During fundholding, practices were actively involved in the planning and commissioning of hospital services. Since that time the Audit Commission recognised that only about 28% of GPs now feel that they have an active role in the commissioning of hospital treatment.

Key factors for the practice to consider

Look back on historic information. What did your practice do during the days of fundholding, if it participated? What sort of model was employed? Was it working on its own or was it part of a bigger group or consortium? Did it get involved in a total purchasing project? By evaluating this, the practice will gain an idea of where a good starting point might be for practice based commissioning. It can learn from its involvement at this stage. Who was involved in the practice? Are these staff and clinicians still working at the practice?

Look at your practice contract, whether GMS or PMS. Particularly with PMS, the practice will already have submitted a business plan. This can form the basis of the practice plan, which can be expanded to include a section on commissioning. Keep things simple and use the resources that have already been developed in the practice. Do not keep re-inventing the wheel. Look at the practice make-up. Does the practice have GPs with specialist interests or GPs who provide sessions already in secondary care? A logical development would be for these practitioners to consider providing these services locally, for both their own patients and for other patients in the area.

One of the restrictions for allowing such services to develop is the availability of space and adequate equipment. However, by carrying out a review of current usage, it may be possible to identify rooms that could be suitably adapted to carry out these services. Also, if the practice is already involved in a project to refurbish, expand or relocate its existing premises, then serious consideration should be given to the potential of future new services being provided in the primary care setting.

The practice should consider the other practices in their immediate vicinity and consider whether it will be of benefit to work with these practices when considering their own plans. Do not forget that the PCT already has a responsibility in respect of public health and public involvement, so early dialogue with the PCT, and ensuring that the practice plans accord with these key principles, is vital.

The introduction of practice based commissioning will inevitably create a period of potential instability. This will be determined locally and understanding the role of the PCT and how the practice is accountable is important. The PCT will be responsible for the implementation locally of the agreed scheme and therefore will be responsible for the management of change. They will be required to engage local clinicians, practice staff and other key stakeholders. They will be responsible for producing systems to effectively monitor the development of services across their area. The practice might ask if the PCT is doing all of this, then why do they need to worry about it. If the practice is not actively involved then the PCT will have failed in one of its basic requirements of engaging clinicians and other staff. To that end some PCTs have devolved staff at local level to represent groups of practices, whereas others have remained committed to a central support team.

The practice might reasonably expect the PCT to be able to provide referral activity by practice, budget support, service level agreement support, guidance on national issues and appropriate training. Already established as part of the overall accountability framework, is the PEC. Understanding what the PEC does will give the practice a clearer view about how they themselves must operate under practice based commissioning.

Key functions

The key functions expected from the PEC are likely to be as follows:

- Form the focal point for the future development of practice based commissioning

- Assist in the development of clear clinical pathways

- Oversee and recommend how savings can be used to fund reasonable management costs

- Check to see that local service level agreements are in place

- Ensure that the whole process remains transparent

- Be responsible for monitoring activity and spend

- Make proposals to the PCT board that take into consideration the contribution made by making changes, the benefits to patients, public health issues, value for money, stakeholder involvement and patient involvement.

Having been advised by the PEC, the PCT board will be responsible for agreeing to any statutory processes, as appropriate. They will ensure that probity and conflict of interest are addressed. Most of all, they have a clear directive to ensure that the general public is clearly involved in the practice based commissioning process.

Table 1: The accountability framework

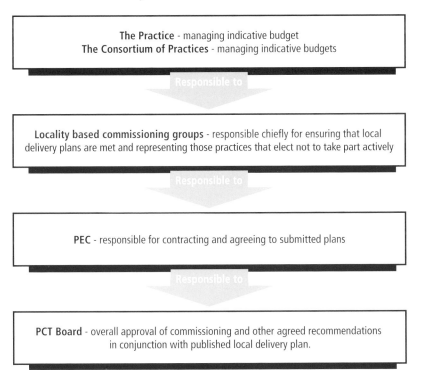

The Practice - managing indicative budget
The Consortium of Practices - managing indicative budgets

Responsible to

Locality based commissioning groups - responsible chiefly for ensuring that local delivery plans are met and representing those practices that elect not to take part actively

Responsible to

PEC - responsible for contracting and agreeing to submitted plans

Responsible to

PCT Board - overall approval of commissioning and other agreed recommendations in conjunction with published local delivery plan.

Having understood the general accountability framework, it will be sensible for the practice to define how it sees itself working in the above structure; without this involvement, there are real dangers that practice based commissioning will not succeed.

Each practice will need to gain an understanding of the wider commissioning agenda within their PCT area by understanding the current local delivery plan. This is not saying that they necessarily agree with the entire plan. However, without at least acknowledging what already exists, it will be difficult to effect their own change. The practice should agree a realistic timescale to implement the new changes. Do not be rail-roaded into agreeing to the first proposal put forward. Take time, reflect and, using local information, make informed decisions.

Some practices are already engaged in good discussions with patients by utilising their own patient participation groups. The QOF has already led to an annual survey, which could be extended to capture information about referrals and hospital services. One problem here is that where the practice does not have a patient participation group, it is required to discuss the results of its survey with a non-executive of the PCT. Recent history has shown that this has not always been possible, which could indicate that there may need to be measures put in place that clearly define what does or does not constitute appropriate involvement of patients and other stakeholders.

To assist at any point, the practice should consider obtaining the views of the local medical committee, who should act as an impartial source and may be able to assist in the event that matters require arbitration.

The PCT will need to be accountable to the local Strategic Health Authority and will be responsible for annual reporting of practice based commissioning in defined demographic areas. They will encourage best practice and share experiences that will be key, given the great diversification that could occur. They will also be responsible for overall arbitration in the event of disputes.

Planning information

The Administrator may be expected to collate or provide data to assist in the planning process.

The Manager will produce interim reports, using currently available financial data. This could include what goods or services are commissioned. They might provide information in relation to practice assets, such as medical equipment or fixtures and fittings.

The Strategist will review service development and undertake asset management reviews. They will be able to advise on what systems should be in place to ensure the appropriate replacement of assets and how and when services could be developed.

Health needs assessment

The Administrator will collect information to assist the process of assessing health needs in the practice.

The Manager will liaise with clinical staff and help to establish a relationship between differing clinical areas, ensuring that all health needs are met.

The Strategist should look at public health issues and look at prevalence factors for the practice. They should be able to look at local demographic issues and will instigate, with clinicians, services to match health needs.

Important: *Using the care pathways described earlier, look at the areas identified and link the practice health needs assessment to the current structure. Take the opportunity to detail future needs, where these are known, e.g. the provision of a new clinic or service.*

> **Advice tip:** When considering a new service think about the extra cost (overheads), workforce and space requirements. These all have an impact on the smooth running of the practice.

Development plans and reports

The Administrator will be responsible for ensuring that the processes required to produce information to support development plans are available and also that the means to produce routine reports is functional. These are the type of reports that might be necessary on a regular basis, such as access figures or number of referrals per month.

The Manager will be able to contribute to development plans and also apply the findings of certain reports and make decisions using this information.

The Strategist will contribute directly to the formulation of development plans and will analyse and make recommendations from the findings of reports. An example of this could be in relation to a service provided by the practice in conjunction with other service organisations, such as a walk-in baby clinic. Proper analysis of reported information would allow a decision to be made about the future frequency or development of the service.

For information: *Produce a list of key development plans and reports together with the report frequency, i.e. monthly, annually, etc.*

Advice tip: Do not produce reports for the sake of it. If a report is read and used then it has a purpose. Collating information that people do not use is unnecessary. If information is requested, ask how it is being used and request feedback.

Strategic delivery planning

The Administrator will understand the process and may assist in the initial planning phase.

The Manager, involving the clinical staff, will review the demographics of the practice and be able to evaluate health need changes for the future. This can be carried out by analysing and interpreting available data.

The Strategist will not only assist in the future direction of the practice but will also look at the financial implications and human resource implications for future changes.

For information: *Consider creating a practice mission statement that reflects concisely where the practice sees itself and what it considers its practice population base to be in the future.*

Advice tip: Start by defining your own statement and then share this with others. It will make it easier to get a mutually agreed definition.

The Effective Manager

1. Attempt to obtain your own practice information about the level of referrals within the practice and record it. Compare this with data provided to you and the information that is used to construct the initial indicative budget. Understand any divergence from the practice information and consider a plan to ensure that the actual activity is properly recorded.

2. Produce a basic PDSA cycle to follow, and then document new PDSA cycles that emerge from the original idea. Good PDSA cycles will generate new cycles. The collection of each of these cycles will provide a documented audit trail of the practice planning process.

3. Wherever possible use the resources that are already at the disposal of the practice. The PMS or GMS contracts already have reporting and monitoring requirements that can be easily adapted to include the aims and objectives for practice based commissioning and reporting accordingly. Being well organised is an essential part of good planning and execution of the same plans.

CHAPTER 4

Negotiating with the PCT

In theory, there should be no need for hard negotiation with the PCT because of the transparency and underlying principles of the commissioning model. What may be more of a problem are the low activity areas or specialist areas that are particular to a small minority of practice patients. Obviously, you will want to negotiate the best for all of your patients, but there will be areas where there will need to be collaborative arrangements in place to satisfy this requirement. This is where the negotiation with the PCT will be important.

This negotiation will almost certainly be underwritten by a basic written agreement, which will stipulate the underlying principles of the level of services to be contracted. It will then be necessary to establish who is responsible for what, making it clear where the responsibilities lie between the PCT and the practice. Remember, it is the practice that is influencing the commissioning decisions, but it is the PCT who still remain responsible for the actual cash flow and administrative support role. This leads onto one obvious area, which is about risk management. It is fine if efficiency savings are identified; the practice will want to be able to influence how this money is re-invested into primary care. Conversely, the practice is less likely to want to underwrite any potential overspends. So risk management (*Appendix B*) is important and a degree of sharing will need to be established.

Having negotiated the contract level with the PCT and having agreed a risk management strategy, it then becomes essential to be able to evaluate the overall service delivery and verify the outcomes.

Effectively, this means ensuring that there is a robust method of audit and evaluation of the selected services.

A new partnership

In order for the commissioning process to work effectively there must be a genuine partnership between the practices and the PCT. The commissioning process should, if effective, demonstrate changes to clinical patterns. Practices are free to work independently or as groups. The latter is preferred by the PCTs because it will mean economies of scale and shared risk management. However, this cannot be imposed on the individual practice, which can still opt to manage a budget on its own. In fact, it goes further than that, because budgets can be devolved to other clinicians such as practice nurses. Community matrons or nurse practitioners could be responsible for patients with long-term illnesses.

At the outset, there needs to be clear dialogue with the PCT in order that both sides understand when there can be an intervention should any key national targets become threatened by commissioning patterns. Should there be any significant deviation away from national targets this could herald the withdrawal of the budget and continuation from being involved in commissioning. With the introduction of patient choice, the commissioning process is vital in ensuring that patients are referred to the right place at the right time. Therefore, practice based commissioning is not just about service level agreements; it is also about the management of referral patterns.

Practices will be expected to review their own referral management styles. Patient choice and the advent of alternative providers, private providers and GPs with special interests mean that there will be a number of alternatives. It is expected that over time these avenues will be expanded upon. The PCT will expect that practices who engage in practice based commissioning also become involved in the choose and book programme. Choose and book and patient choice means that there are additional factors that must be agreed between the PCT and practice.

If the PCT already has existing agreements in place with different agencies or trusts, the practices will be expected to honour such agreements and ensure that the practice plans reflect those agreements. Where there are fine divisions between who are provider and commissioner, it is important that a conflict of interest is not created. It will be important to establish probity in respect of the use of public funds. To that end practices, in conjunction with the PCT, will expect the involvement of local community groups and patients in the planning process. The PCT are duty bound by the Health and Social Care Act 2001 to ensure that this element is carried out.

Patient choice

What also needs to be negotiated with the PCT is the principle of how patients may exercise choice. It is not just about choosing the provider, but also the choice of not using the practice if it is the provider. There must be no pressure put on the patients. In future, patients may be given the opportunity of choosing more than one practice to gain access to the optimum level of services.

It is becoming clear that involving patients and allowing them to exercise their right to patient choice will mean that there will be a significant number of interested parties. There are three scenarios that could be faced locally:

Scenario 1 - No real demand from patients or other stakeholders. Practice based commissioning continues almost as it currently operates

Scenario 2 - Patients and stakeholders request specific changes to current service provision

Scenario 3 - Patients and stakeholders disagree entirely with the local delivery plan and want to change everything.

In reality, it is likely to be a combination of all scenarios that must be effectively managed over time. The practice should be prepared to negotiate with the PCT over numerous issues. It must also be aware that in the event that matters cannot be mutually resolved, there is an arbitration process. In order to make sure that it has a good case to be heard, the practice needs to ensure that throughout the process it has considered the following key points:

Table 2: Consideration points for negotiating with PCT

The practice perspective	
Has the practice	• Considered strategic importance?
	• Recognised PCT objectives?
	• Managed to improve patient care?
The budget	• What scope of budget is held?
Status	• Is this a single practice or a group?
Proposal	• Is the proposal clearly defined and is there clinical structure in place to support it?
The PCT perspective	
Proposal	• Why was the proposal rejected?
Strategy	• Has the strategy been discussed at PEC/Board level?
GPs	• Can local involvement be demonstrated?

The above lists are not exhaustive, but give a flavour of how either side might fail to win in the event of arbitration. It also shows that there would need to be a complete breakdown of local implementation to necessitate arbitration in the first place.

When negotiating with the PCT, the practice needs to be strong and ensure that its views are heard. However, it must also be realistic and accept that there may be competing needs, which means the prioritisation of certain service developments over others. A sensible timescale is also important. Services must be allowed to develop and not simply be imposed. Proper evaluation of any changes should be undertaken and reviewed.

Working partnership

The Administrator must ensure that they know the practice's key stakeholders and ensure that there is a good rapport established. Primarily this will include the PCO and their staff.

The Manager will extend this role to include external organisations and may be responsible for arranging meetings, or establishing better relationships, with these groups.

The Strategist should be at the leading edge when it comes to fostering existing or new working relationships. They will consider any areas where there might be gaps or where there are too many contacts. They can advise on how best to address these and produce a framework of associated personnel that can best serve the practice needs.

For information: *Produce a list of key stakeholders. Wherever possible cross-reference this to other areas of the competency framework. This will avoid duplication of effort.*

Advice tip: Obtain the email addresses of the key contacts, even if you do not need to contact them on a regular basis. Be ready for the time that you do.

Networking with other practices

The Administrator should be aware of local contacts and try to network with them during training or monthly practice meetings. Normally these are organised by the responsible PCO.

The Manager should oversee local relationships and consider the fostering of new relationships. This can lead to the avoidance of the duplication of effort if a neighbouring practice is able to share information or resources.

The Strategist will look at gaps within its own practice and try to identify local knowledge that could be utilised. Other managers will very often happily provide assistance or support or, more importantly, share their own experiences.

For information: *Produce a list of areas that you feel might help the practice and try to identify local resources that could assist in the future. For example, you might want to meet with other managers and ask them for their own areas of expertise and record this for future use.*

Advice tip: Once you have networked with other managers, stay in contact and help each other out. Again this is an area where email is very useful.

Liaison with other care providers

These providers are mainly hospitals providing secondary care and tertiary providers, which could be specialist units or community services and the voluntary sector.

The Administrator should be able to ensure that there are effective communication systems in place between providers. Chiefly this will include initial point of contact, but can include the provision of information to assist in problem areas or to improve services.

The Manager can act as a contact point in the event of the absence of the GP and will be able to enact changes to improve communication at their own discretion.

The Strategist will identify where the weaknesses are and can initiate the discussion for a mutual resolution. This can be a sensitive area at times because of the differing operational requirements of each organisation, and therefore it requires diplomacy and patience when considering making changes.

For information: *Produce a list of key contacts and telephone numbers or emails, in particular those that relate to practice referrals. Consider the use of a communication flowchart so that everyone can see at a glance who the key stakeholders are.*

> **Advice tip:** Consider the use of at least one letter per year, updating your stakeholders with your practice information and inviting them to update you with any of their changes.

The Effective Manager

1. Identify the lead persons in the PCT responsible for the commissioning process. Establish the basis of communication with these people. Ask for a copy of the local delivery plan.

2. Identify the lead persons in the local providers and establish the communication links with these organisations. Try to obtain information about prices, waiting times and location of services.

3. Speak to the PCT and get a clear understanding of the local agenda for meeting the requirements of patient choice. This will identify the key providers, which will be useful in assessing the practice's own commissioning agenda.

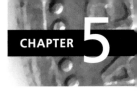

CHAPTER 5

Management costs

As ever, management costs could become a contentious issue, if there is not a clear understanding from the outset of what is reasonable and what is not. In fundholding, there was a clearly defined allowance available for practices to work within. This sum was audited annually, hence fulfilling all the aspects discussed previously. Namely, risk management, audit and evaluation.

Management input and/or support is crucial to achieving a successful commissioning model. The potential costs will need to be agreed with the PCT in advance and subsequently offset against efficiency gains arising from changed clinical patterns.

What will probably happen is that the PCT will issue a policy detailing how practices may bid to recover management costs from the resources that may become available at the end of the year. It is likely that there will be a local process that is open and transparent for all practices to be given equal access to recover such costs. Management costs can cover a variety of areas, so it may be prudent for joint arrangements to be put in place for areas such as finance, IT and clinical governance issues.

Typical costs

What are going to be the most likely additional costs to be faced by practices that may be claimable as management costs?

- Doctor A decides to become more involved in the commissioning process and decides to become part of the steering group for a group of practices exploring joint commissioning. He or she will need to spend time attending meetings and discussing issues with colleagues. Therefore, this time can be paid for by allowing the appropriate reimbursement of locum costs, whilst the doctor is undertaking these new duties.

■ The practice will want to keep a record of its own referral patterns and be able to substantiate this with paid activity. This will increase the workload of existing administrative or data staff within the practice.

■ Continuing professional development, training and conferences will be available. GPs and staff will need time to attend events and therefore arrangements will need to be put in place to cover the cost of events and reimburse the cost of paying other staff or locums to carry out existing duties whilst absent from work.

■ Instead of using existing staff or GP time, it may be better to appoint specialist support and utilise this time efficiently. There may be possibilities to operate weighted capitation or local equivalents to ensure equity of costs.

■ There are ultimately going to be costs associated with IT capital costs and administration, and software to support commissioning arrangements. It will be the responsibility of the PCT to meet these costs, but with limited resources, they are likely to want to procure such equipment as reasonable costs offset against management costs.

Local developments – a health warning

As there is no current robust commissioning framework, commissioning will be allowed to develop at a local level. The costs of developing services, including implementation, audit and research, will be classed as reasonable costs.

However, there is a health warning associated with management costs. Wherever possible, practices and PCTs are expected to utilise the skills of existing commissioning staff. Do not forget that if you were involved in fundholding commissioning or locality based commissioning then you are likely to possess the basic skills for use in the current commissioning framework. Be aware that we are now in an era of cash limited budgets. PCTs are already facing large overspends, which basically will not be resolved over one financial year. As a result of this there may be a danger that funds could be top-sliced by the PCT hoping that any resulting efficiencies will fund future management costs.

Assuming that it is possible to identify savings, the decision of how much may be spent on management costs lies within the remit of the Professional Executive Committee. The PEC will want to ensure that there are shared arrangements, particularly with regard to public health issues, finance and IT.

Rewarding the practice

As a practice you must be realistic from the outset about what actually constitutes the additional costs to be faced by the practice as a result of entering practice based commissioning. Early discussion needs to be held and agreements reached about what level of costs will be reimbursed. One of the approaches suggested is to reimburse GPs for their time to ensure sufficient clinical input into the process. It is felt that if GPs are involved in validating the data aspect, then in the longer term it will be easier to introduce indicative budgets based on this verified work.

The biggest risk lies in developing good management structures that are actually rewarded for the work that they do. This means at the very least recognising the actual management costs that will be incurred by the practice. The real danger is that although the initial funding will be supported by the PCT, it is on the basis that over a period of time these costs will be self-funding from efficiency savings made year on year.

This is one unknown area, and where this commissioning model varies significantly from the management allowance, which was part of the fundholding scheme.

The main concern for the practice is to ensure that it can identify the true associated costs. If the practice does not incur any additional costs as a result of engaging in practice based commissioning, then the chances are that it is not actively engaged in the process.

Will there be incentives?

If there is doubt about how additional practice costs are to be funded, and if these costs are to be funded from future efficiency savings, then what incentives will be left and where will the funding be for these incentives? This area, which will be determined locally, will probably ultimately have a crucial influence on how practice based commissioning actually develops over time. If there are not the incentives built in above and beyond the basic management costs, it is likely that practices will not feel sufficiently financially encouraged to participate.

Added to this scenario is the possibility that existing funds will be top-sliced to provide a central contingency fund to help manage local risk. Whilst risk management is an important part of any commissioning strategy, it will place an increased demand on available resources for funding local incentives.

It looks as though it will be difficult to identify how incentives will be achieved. With so many PCTs contending with brought-forward deficits it is unlikely with top-slicing and reduced referral rates, that significant additional funds will be realised to fund incentives.

The Effective Manager

1. Firstly, consider who in the clinical team, including nurses, is going to be involved in the process. Detail the number of hours they are involved in practice based commissioning activity; by calculating this and multiplying by the individual's hourly rate, a practice can ascertain the reimbursement that might be expected.

2. Secondly, apply the same process as above to management time. In reality, if a manager is asked to go to a meeting, it means that they are not doing their normal daily tasks. Very rarely will they be replaced by a locum manager; this then becomes a hidden cost for the practice.

3. Lastly, do not forget general support staff, whether secretaries or data clerks, receptionists and general admin. Support staff are always helping clinicians and managers, and their time must be costed. An effective manager will delegate responsibilities to support staff, so it will be inevitable that these additional costs will be incurred.

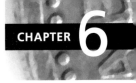

The commissioning budget

Where do you start? There is to be no national model; instead the budget-setting model is to be based around local solutions. How much you become involved will depend on each practice. The whole process is voluntary. However, if a practice does not feel the process that has been agreed locally is allowing them enough involvement, they can request an indicative budget for the full range of services.

Although guidance has been issued to assist in budget setting, it may be that there is local agreement to await the availability of 2004/05 data about actual service levels.

The principles of the commissioning model mean that a practice will hold an indicative budget for the full range of patient services, ensuring that all commissioned care is covered. This means that there will be services beyond the scope of the national tariff and consequently local decisions about costs will need to be made.

Key budget setting principles

What are the basic principles that will underpin a budget setting methodology? The following are a few of the key principles that must be included in the process:

- The whole process needs to be transparent

- The process must be sympathetic to the existing health needs

- Will need to refer to historical data

- Will not be allowed to exceed the PCT cash-limited overall budget

- Should be a simple process to begin with and developed over time

- Should compare local data against national tariff rates, where published

- Support the development of enhanced services and achievement of local targets

- Should ensure that there are no service inequalities - this way no one can complain of a two-tier service

- Should allow for contingencies or significant changes of activity

- Should ensure that adequate risk management is assessed and appropriate strategies developed.

Given the above, the budgets still need to be sufficiently flexible to allow incentives to be built in, which encourage innovative implementation or the redesign of services. Practices will want to make contributions to the process in the knowledge that there will be a reasonable return for the effort needed to create the efficiencies. There is no doubt that a fluid practice population, either a growing or reducing list size, will affect an individual practice's budget. A simple process of defining list sizes needs to be agreed locally and then implemented accordingly. This process could be annual, monthly or at any other agreed time interval.

Those services that are covered by the national tariff will be relatively easy to calculate using existing historical data. Those not covered by this tariff will need to be agreed locally. At the moment, these services are covered by the PCT and it is likely that they will remain outside the initial budget setting discussions, with contracts being managed by the PCT.

The approach for 2005/06

The Department of Health has shown strong support for local deter-mination of indicative budgets during 2005/06. The technical guid-ance that has been issued is so flexible that undoubtedly a variety of local models will be created. Technical guidance is designed to allow a default budget to be allocated, in case a practice opts to claim the right to a commissioning budget that covers a full range of patient services. During 2005/06, this is restricted to elective in-patient and day case treatment only, for which the national tariff will apply. First wave Foundation Trusts *(see Appendix E)* will use the tariff for 2005/06 for non-elective in-patient treatment, all outpatient appointments, and accident and emergency activity.

Understanding your budget

Hospital Episode Statistics (HES) will be averaged for 2003/04 and allocated into groups of practices. These will form the share to be allocated in the first instance. Importance in the process is placed on changes to list sizes and local adjustments for services that may already be incorporated into the local delivery plan. The technical process is explained later, but this chapter looks at some of the anomalies that might arise as a result of a locally introduced scheme.

HES data for 2003/04 will contain errors, which could potentially destabilise the budgetary process. It is believed that up to 2% of data could contain inaccuracies or simply be incorrectly coded. 2% may not seem a lot on a global basis, but will have a more significant impact at individual practice level.

Any uplift applied from 2003/04 to 2005/06 will need to take account of the forecast level of activity for 2005/06. This is key because as a result of Foundation Trusts being established, these organisations have now started achieving activity levels that are above what was originally planned. The incentive for this has been that they believe they will be funded as per the payment by results programme.

Little spoken about, but as important to understanding your budget, is not just the move of services between secondary and primary care or the use of other providers, but is also the setting of contingency plans and planned savings strategies. In lots of cases, it simply has not been possible to move forward the commissioning process, other than by establishing working groups for 2005/06. There is also a real danger that no real progress will be made during 2006/07, because there still need to be discussions about the local delivery plan. In reality, what has already been agreed with providers within the local delivery plan may not fit seamlessly with practices' own intentions, and it may take a couple of years to progress to a definitive indicative budget that truly reflects the plans of the practice.

It has already been mentioned that the historical methodology of funding practice based commissioning will give rise to unfair shares of funds being distributed between practices. This is designed to be equalised by 2006/07, but the only practice not to be affected by this style of funding will be the practice that is truly at the average level for its current list size. Given this scenario, the practice must make early representations if there are specific reasons why they might not be considered an average practice. For example, if a practice serves a higher than average number of residential or nursing homes, this will need to be addressed.

The core competency framework has many expected degrees of competency aimed at financial management. These are summarised below:

Resource allocation

The Administrator should have a basic understanding of how the practice is funded and the principles of equity. This should include an understanding of top-down funding and cash-limited budgets.

The Manager will look at the overall resources available and check these against current expenditure being offset against it. By understanding at a local level the competing demands against resources, it is possible to make fact-based decisions.

The Strategist will be aware of the funding model being used and will assess this funding model with regard to the needs of the practice. They should also assess any other sources of funding and any other models that could be more favourable for the practice.

Monthly accounting

The Administrator can be involved in basic record keeping and could be involved in the production of data, under supervision, for the purposes of producing monthly management accounts.

The Manager will be responsible for ensuring that accounting data is properly entered into manual or computer records. They will be able to reconcile information, including the monthly reconciliation statement. They will be able to introduce accounting systems and to produce management reports in the form of simple statements.

The Strategist will have an understanding of accounting techniques and advise on the format of the monthly management accounts. They will advise staff how to operate systems and how to collate data. They can be responsible for undertaking any necessary training.

For information: *Produce a monthly management finance report. Do not make this too detailed or it will be cumbersome to use. Keep it simple, but make it consistent. Simple indicators, normally in the form of financial variances, should be sufficient to indicate problem areas and allow remedial action to be taken.*

> **Advice tip:** Initially look only at the larger variances, and then over a period of time you should see the level of variance decrease, which should save time in monitoring the reports.

Service budgets

The Administrator is not involved in this area.

The Manager will manage devolved budgets under the supervision of the GP or the Strategist and take responsibility for how delegated sums are spent. This can be done at times without supervision.

The Strategist should take overall responsibility for allocating individual service budgets and ensure that adequate probity is maintained with the person responsible for managing the budget. They will be able to be involved in practice training issues.

For information: *Keep service budgets simple - in other words, only allocate sums for specific requirements. Do not over-complicate issues.*

Advice tip: Do not devolve budgets unnecessarily. If you do devolve a budget ensure that the person to whom it is delegated understands the implications of any over- or underspending.

Resource negotiation

The Administrator could be involved in the discussion of how resources are used to develop practice services and support their use.

The Manager will have a greater understanding of resource implications and will be able to report on this from time to time. They will be able to initiate discussions with the PCO on resource issues relating to the practice programme of patient care.

The Strategist will undertake the responsibility of producing a practice business case for the PCO that identifies the financial requirements to fulfil the practice programme of care for its patients.

For information: *Consider what the practice wants to do for its patient population in the future and produce a synopsis of a business case. Work up this synopsis into a full business case at the appropriate time.*

> **Advice tip:** Keep this very concise and to the point. However, do amend it to reflect current thinking and, as with the above, use it when appropriate to develop a stronger business case when competing for restricted resources.

The Effective Manager

1. Always have to hand a summary of how the indicative budget is made up, together with an audit trail of how the initial costs have been funded. Then try to establish where the practice is in comparison with a weighted capitation form of funding. This is important, particularly if the practice is historically above the local average.

2. Consider the format of a monthly management report, which can be used to see actual cost against budget, but also identify referral fluctuations. Linking this report to the published waiting times allows you very quickly to start to predict projected overspends or underspends by speciality.

3. Identify all those patients that fall into the category of six-month choice. These are patients that are likely to exceed the six-month waiting time. These patients will be offered the choice of attending another provider, which could lead to additional costs. These costs should be assessed, because they could have an impact on the final value of savings achieved. Conversely, if the cost of the alternative provider proves to be cheaper, this could influence the choice of providers in the future.

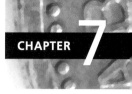

CHAPTER 7

Information technology

Data is the key to developing a robust commissioning system. If the data is bad, the output will also be of poor quality. Therefore, it is imperative that work be done at the earliest opportunity to ensure sound data collection. History has proven that there can be a wide variation between what practices say is happening and what providers say is happening. Although this will be critical in informing early discussions and may contribute to early budget setting models, as time goes on and payment by results becomes mainstream, there will be less emphasis put on this initial data.

The PCT will act as a conduit to provide data to practices, which in turn may have their own information sources for comparison or audit purposes. At the moment PCTs will provide information to practices about usage of services. To make commissioning work effectively, information needs to be timely and accurate. This information also needs to be reviewed on a regular basis.

Whatever system is adopted, it will need to address the following key areas:

1. Data accuracy and timeliness

2. Patient profiles to assist risk management

3. Adaptability to clinical change

4. Cost targeting

5. Patient uptake and appropriate usage

6. Manage demand (remember patient choice and choose and book)

7. Clear audit trails of data.

Practices should look at their own existing clinical systems and see how these can be used to validate their patient activity, whatever type of referral has been made.

A universal IT solution

The Department of Health has not as yet made a definite commitment to how practice based commissioning will be supported from an information technology point of view. Many PCTs and local providers have already developed their own activity capture software. However, in some cases, the providers have good systems and the PCTs have little or no systems in place. In these cases, there is ongoing dialogue about the ownership and use of the data. The initial software available will assist in developing the financial aspect and allow the indicative budgets to be allocated.

The Department of Health is engaged in ongoing work to evaluate the IT requirements to support this initiative. It should be remembered that the final resolution to this scheme would result in a variety of options to integrate with the providers' and PCTs' existing IT solutions. These may be valuable to the overall process, but in the longer term it is envisaged that these systems will be adapted or built upon to eventually provide a firm foundation for future commissioning software programmes. This is not to say that existing systems will be subsumed, unlike fundholding, where accredited software was effectively committed ineffectual overnight, following the abolition of the scheme.

PCTs will be encouraged to work with providers to develop data solutions utilising the best parts of existing systems. Local providers will keep detailed records of all activity and these should form the core of any validated data. However, it is known that there is a percentage error of data held, which will need to be improved upon over time.

Utilising the payments by results system connected to a national tariff should mean a definite and definable link between actual activity and cost. The introduction of patient choice and the choose and book initiative will mean that more and more activity information regarding referral activity will be available at the same level entry point.

Data collection

The Department of Health has three or four different systems for collating national data, which could be modified to assist in the process. The prescription pricing authority has been successfully using a system that links cost and activity for many years, and has been feeding this information back to practices; practice based commissioning should follow a similar pattern. The introduction of the QOF has educated practices in the management of activity information and related this to cost. This will be important for assisting in the introduction of any cost/activity related system. There is still continuing work being done on QOF data, which could be extended to assist in the commissioning model.

A variety of PCTs have already developed their own methodologies for addressing the initial IT needs. Whilst not without their own levels of risk, these schemes have been evaluated and the observations will be collated by the primary care contracting team. This is one of the NHS' specialist teams set up to evaluate and deal with developments in primary care contracting. These local initiatives are likely to be supported in conjunction with a national IT strategy and support network.

The IT plan

The plan is at least to have the financial systems in place by January 2006 to assist in ensuring the process of practice based commissioning can be implemented from April 2006. In the meantime, if a PCT is considering proceeding with developing its own local solutions, it needs to ensure the following criteria are addressed:

- Will practices be informed of their indicative budgets as individual practices or as a group?

- Can this budget be broken down?

- With what frequency will the PCT provide details of costed activity to practices?

- Where does this activity data come from?

- What is the basis of the costing of this activity?

- Has the data been fully verified?

- Is all activity captured, including primary care and other providers?

- Do practices provide their own electronic data?

- How are data transferred to or from the practice and what is the source?

- Are the existing practice clinical systems or separate sub-systems used?

- How do commissioners use information to request the PCT to act?

- Does the PCT actually act upon requests from practitioners?

- Can the PCT produce any performance reports for practices?

When you look at the above, there is a potential risk that some areas will develop quicker than others and that might destabilise the full implementation of practice based commissioning in some areas. Although there has not yet been much information published regarding how data will be captured, exchanged or shared, the practice should continue to develop its own level of competencies in accordance with how it manages its existing contract and the QOF.

Data management

The Administrator will be able to input and retrieve referral data for reporting purposes.

The Manager will be able to do the above, but will also be able to initiate practice audits or ad hoc searches for data. They can provide training to junior staff.

The Strategist will oversee the management of data within the practice and should look at which information is retrieved regularly from the computer system and how this information is used.

For information: *Draw up a list of regular reports run by the practice including the quality and outcomes searches, and detail the frequency of when the reports are run.*

Advice tip: Analyse the data produced by the practice and if information is not used, then do not produce it.

Data security

The Administrator will ensure that they know the security systems utilised within the practice and who has what access to what system.

The Manager will consider the statutory requirements and will be familiar with data protection issues. Primarily this will include the Data Protection Act and the Access to Information Act in respect of deceased patients. The manager will understand the complexities of data exchange between parties.

The Strategist will be conversant with NHSnet issues and guidelines and will ensure that the practice systems comply accordingly.

Important: *Ensure that the practice documents the key issues identified in the NHSnet guidelines.*

Advice tip: If the use of email is provided to staff, ensure that this medium is used for appropriate purposes, and in particular ensure that patient confidentiality is not compromised.

Data interpretation and manipulation

The Administrator will be able to collect, import and export the data in a suitable format for use with other applications.

The Manager will be able to do the above and also be able to report on the outcomes. They will be able to analyse this data and comment on practice performance.

The Strategist will undertake full analysis and review of data. They will evaluate the effects of the data on practice performance. They can help develop reporting formats or even prepare templates for practice use.

For information: *If the practice develops its own templates or reports, detail the systems used and why the reports are needed.*

Advice tip: Review any practice templates and identify why and by whom they are used. Is all the information relevant? Templates can duplicate effort if the people using them do not understand how the information is stored within the computer system.

The Effective Manager

1. Use your existing clinical system to collate existing referral information. These clinical systems use a variety of read codes that can be searched accordingly. You will be surprised how much information is already available.

2. Use new innovations. For example, if you are already in the process of implementing choose and book, consider the information that can be taken from this new scheme.

3. In the event that there is a paucity of information initially, remember that the practice already writes referral letters. This information is readily available, can be attached to the clinical system and easily reported on. Hopefully, the new software developed for commissioning will resolve this matter; however, during fundholding, software was developed that would write the referral letter which would be automatically recorded. If many practices were asked they would admit that they still get their own referral letters typed.

CHAPTER 8

How savings are spent

Savings or efficiency gains may seem more attractive with the tag that 100% may be used by the practice for the development and implementation of patient services. However, all is not what it might seem. Unlike fundholding, where there were specific criteria for the use of savings, any efficiency gains achieved under practice based commissioning will be subject to many external influences.

The savings that are produced will be net of any management costs. Any subsequent spending will need to receive approval from the PCT. So what will the PCT be likely to approve? Practices and the PCT will be able to look at referral patterns and explore how waiting times could be reduced by using more appropriately placed practitioners. Consultant led clinics in a primary care setting is not a new idea, but it is one that has proven to be both successful and popular. With the added requirement of wider patient choice, the system adopted will need to be both proactive and reactive to such demands. Existing care pathways *(Appendix A)* may need to be re-visited and even completely re-designed.

So, the plan is to deliver a service that allows the patient to benefit from a greater range of services, from a greater number of providers, in locations more convenient to them. Having delivered this plan, the practice can benefit from the efficiencies achieved unless, say, the PCT has a large financial deficit to contend with. Initial funding of primary care commissioning will be underwritten by the PCT, who will be entitled to recoup these funds from any early efficiency gains. It may not be possible to enjoy the rewards of the scheme in the early years due to these cost pressures. In many regional variations, schemes have been implemented to account for these early discrepancies. What is clear is that it is vital that the mechanism to achieve efficiency gains is apparent and that any external cost pressures are transparent from the outset. Otherwise, the result could be a lot of effort undertaken at practice level, with little potential for achieving true efficiency gains. Practices could end up becoming the conduit to resolving PCTs' financial problems.

Planning the use of savings

Assuming that it has been possible to achieve savings and additional management costs have been met, there will be a sum available for re-investment into patient services. Included in this could be the investment in capital projects that will allow expanded services to be delivered in the future. Part of the planning process will be the declaration at the beginning of the financial year on how such savings will be applied. This will receive approval at the outset following approval by the PEC. Where there are disputes, the locally agreed arbitration process will apply. There may be occasions where there becomes a conflict of interest, caused by the membership structure of the PEC. In these instances, declarations of interest will need to be made to ensure transparency at all times. When deciding what proposals should be agreed by the PCT board, the following issues need to be accommodated:

- The impact any proposals make to key NHS framework targets and the overall financial status of the PCT

- The benefits to patients

- Risk is minimised, but innovation and new ideas are allowed to be experimented with

- There will be demonstrable healthcare gains

- Value for money is achieved and the healthcare provided is appropriate

- Plans ensure there is full agreement amongst all stakeholders

- All key staff are allowed to influence the decisions.

Unlike fundholding, where a management allowance was paid up front, under practice based commissioning, any funding for efficiencies or reasonable management costs have to be funded initially by the PCT, but ultimately recouped from the overall indicative budget. PCTs have, therefore, played down the level of incentives that might be achieved. However, they have had to ensure that they have not dampened the enthusiasm of practices too much or there will be a danger that the whole process will simply not work.

The PCT will need to make it transparent how incentive payments will be made and at what frequency. The types of initiatives that they are likely to support will be those areas that practices have indicated that they are keen to participate in; those initiatives that will provide a benefit to the practice on a day-to-day basis. The following areas have been widely recognised as being areas that can be commissioned and will allow the kind of incentives to be gained that will assist in keeping practices actively engaged:

Table 3: Popular areas for commissioning

General surgery	Elderly care
Orthopaedics	Mental health
Urology	Teenage pregnancy
Oral surgery	Minor surgery
Ophthalmology	Most outpatient appointments
ENT	

The above list is just an example and as the scheme continues, and payment by results becomes more mainstream then, in theory, all specialities should become equalised.

One thing is certain; if appropriate incentive arrangements are put in place, then the practice will show greater willingness to participate and make an active contribution to the process. Without the right level of incentives, the speed at which a practice will actively engage in the process will clearly be delayed. PCTs will need to publish at an early stage what types of incentives might be available. This might be initially difficult where PCTs have to contend with brought-forward overspends.

If a practice wants to evaluate how likely it will be to achieve sufficient incentives under the scheme, it may need to make an assessment on how it feels its responsible PCT will be ready to embrace the commissioning process.

Table 4: What the practice should consider

1. What is the current relationship with the PCT?

2. Does the PCT support practice management involvement or does it impose its own management support?

3. Does the PCT have a dedicated commissioning team?

4. Has the PCT provided the practice with details of the local delivery plan and given suggestions of how this plan could be varied?

5. Has it published a clear working paper with regard to budget setting and allocation?

6. Consider how the PCT has managed the QOF process and the level (or lack) of support to achieving maximum payments under the scheme

7. Do they readily make available quality data to the practice and have they got an IT solution in place for practice based commissioning?

8. Have they defined what management support is available, and when, to the practice?

9. Has the PCT got robust monitoring processes in place, meaning it will be possible to identify any efficiencies gained more readily?

Conversely, the practice will need to be able to demonstrate that it has certain levels of competencies, in order for the PCT to be happy to endorse any savings made. The savings must be seen as being planned and deliberately achieved, and not fortuitous.

Minimum practice requirements

Most of the criteria necessary have been mentioned earlier in this book, but the key requirements are repeated here. If the practice can show that they meet these criteria, then any savings achieved will certainly not be fortuitous. Practices should demonstrate the following:

- There is a local delivery plan in place that the practice subscribes to

- The objectives set are realistic and the level of savings aspired to is sensible

- There are no serious contractual issues

- They are adequate QOF performers

- They have adequate IT systems in place

- There are no outstanding disputes with the PCT, such as PMS/GMS contract disputes or high levels of patient complaints

- Patient involvement has been demonstrated

- They are developing systems for patient choice and the introduction of choose and book

- They have clinical governance arrangements in place

- They have an agreement in place with the PCT.

Without any of the above, it is unlikely that the PCT will consider that the practice, or group of practices, have the appropriate infrastructure to be able to make savings.

The Effective Manager

1. Make sure that the practice is up to speed. Ensure that they do not have anything outstanding with the PCT. If the practice is failing to meet contract objectives or is a poor QOF performer, then any savings that might be achieved will come under greater scrutiny and may not be perceived as being planned.

2. Draw up a savings plan and remain committed to it. If the practice is achieving what it has set out to do, then ensure that there is a regular dialogue with the PCT and advise them at an early stage what the practice intends to do with the savings.

3. Be aware of the contribution the practice might have to make towards any deficit brought forward by the PCT. This could have an impact on the level of savings that could be achieved in the first year.

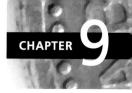

Getting ready

Now that we know that the practice wishes to explore the way services are currently delivered, how does it go about making that change happen? Firstly, it must have a clear understanding of how commissioning currently operates.

The cycle currently adopted within the NHS falls along the following broad outline. During April to September, health needs of local populations are evaluated, which in turn leads to a definition of service requirements for patient populations. From September to November, initial commissioning plans are drawn up and discussions with providers about service delivery or re-design are undertaken. During December to February, contract negotiations are undertaken. Throughout the year, on a monthly and quarterly basis, contracts are monitored. At the end of each year, there should be an evaluation of the services contracted in the previous period, which will then inform the following year's contract programme.

Health needs assessments will reveal what is typically required from one locality to another. Typically, the PCT will have historical data about local health needs. However, local knowledge or actual experience from the practice will be important at the early part of any future planning phase. The practice must consider various issues before even starting to plan future services. The practice should consider the following:

Table 5: Initial planning and considerations

- For the existing practice population (whether an individual practice or a group of practices), does the practice feel happy with the current level of services offered?

- Which services are acceptable and therefore do not need immediate change?

- Of the services that need to be changed, which have the highest priority? Do not forget that the changes required may not just be for financial reasons; they may be due to quality issues or simply about how easy it is to access a particular service

- The practice needs to be realistic about how quickly and how much a service is changed or re-defined. Doing too much too soon could actually have detrimental effects. However, not doing enough will allow an inefficient service to continue unnecessarily

- The practice should make its intentions clear for both the short and long term. It has a responsibility to assist those involved in the commissioning cycle by being explicit about how it sees the future of the provision of hospital based services

- The contract model adopted will need to be sensitive to patient choice and therefore provide referral options in all cases, except where specialist treatment is required. This means that the commissioning model chosen will need to be flexible and adaptable to changing local needs.

As previously stated, prioritising work is important. Neither providers nor the PCT will welcome a large divergence from existing arrangements, and in setting priorities it will be important to ensure that the following are adhered to:

- Consider the service delivery under the terms of the current national service framework and any current guidance issued

- Consider the local development plan of the PCT

- Take on board the views of patients; patient choice will not be effective if the views of patients are ignored

- It must be realistic. This realism is dictated by the current allocation of resources and the fact that there are a number of areas where there are clear deficits in the resources available

- The services chosen must be able to accommodate the principles of choose and book

- The service level agreements will need to take account of public health and clinical governance arrangements.

How will the practice be assessed?

As with all areas of practice based commissioning, there is a distinct lack of precise instructions regarding what must or must not be done. Therefore, in the first instance, it will be best to open up dialogue with the PCT and identify how they wish the practice to proceed. Many PCTs have already set up working groups or locality based commissioning groups who meet to discuss the implementation of the local agenda.

The initial application

It is likely that the basic requirement of the practice will be to submit a local application detailing their own plans in order that these can be reviewed against the overall local delivery plan. Once this has been assessed, a service agreement can be produced which stipulates:

- Clear aims and objectives

- Who the agreement relates to (important when dealing with groups of practices)

- The key services to be commissioned and provided under the agreement

- Accountability and termination details

- The use of data and quality issues

- Performance management (under- or over-performance against agreed targets)

- Contract monitoring and reporting

- Financial management

- Respective roles and responsibilities

- In the case of group practices, any inter-practice agreements explaining roles and responsibilities.

Perhaps an easier way of looking at the process is to consider it as being an addendum to the existing PMS or GMS contract and be prepared to implement and report on the outcomes in a similar fashion. In preparing for the new initiative, consider areas where the practice is already demonstrating levels of competency.

Strategy formulation

The Administrator will be able to provide data for strategic planning and could be available to assist in review and analysis. The data will be collated by utilising reporting systems of the practice medical computer system or asking other members of staff to provide details of work undertaken on a regular basis. An example of this might be to provide details of the number of registered patients on a monthly basis compared with the number of average consultations per GP each month, and then compare this to the number of referrals.

The Manager will be able to discuss the results of the data and liaise with the GP to help assist the management process, discussing the findings and implementing any changes to the number of consultations and workload of individual clinicians.

The Strategist will take it one step further and look at future resource needs in comparison with the number of consultations being held and the resulting referrals. The length of contracts and the use of locums will need to be reviewed and appropriate action taken.

For information: *Devise your own practice management information report. Design the report to be used internally by the practice and keep the information relevant and concise.*

> **Advice tip:** When considering your own practice strategy formulation, highlight any areas that make your practice unique or different from others, and then build the more general planning aspects around this.

Innovation

The Administrator should take part in the feasibility of innovative ideas and will take part in meetings or discussions about ideas put forward. There need not be regular meetings, but opportunities should be made available to staff to contribute ideas.

The Manager will assist the administrator, but is more likely to assess and implement any innovation and report on its evaluation and effectiveness. Remember, some ideas could be tried and will work, others might need to be refined, and some will prove not to be suitable. The principle of innovation is to encourage development and improvements to existing services and procedures. The manager should encourage the active involvement of patients in this area.

The Strategist is likely to be constantly innovating and introducing new ideas. One of the biggest problems they face is that they are perceived by others to be always making the changes and therefore the innovation may be seen as a directive being forced upon others, rather than a new idea that should be adopted by everyone. The strategists need to be sensitive to this fact and introducing an ideas forum and utilising other members of the management team will help facilitate this.

For information: *Develop a forum to promote innovative ideas. Record all ideas and where implemented identify when and how this change benefited the practice.*

> **Advice tip:** List three innovative ideas for the practice. Do this on your own and without input from anyone else. This will help promote genuine innovation. Then share your ideas and evaluate them accordingly.

The Effective Manager

1. Use a checklist like the one shown in Appendix G, to detail the requirements of the practice. Identify who within the practice will be involved in the process and ensure that they are briefed accordingly.

2. Consider at an early stage how the practice will engage the input of patients into the process. If there is already a patient participation group, this would be an ideal forum to carry out the consultation process. If one does not exist, consider using a survey or selecting a quorum of patients (maybe five or six) who could be consulted on an individual basis.

3. Carry out your own risk analysis for the practice. Be aware at the outset of the potential costs to the practice in respect of staff involvement. There are so many initiatives being undertaken by practice staff at the moment that the introduction of this scheme means that resources could be stretched or other areas suffer inadvertently.

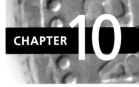

CHAPTER 10

The management phase

Having received an indicative budget, it is vital that it is correctly monitored. Many PCOs already have large overspends to worry about. They will not look favourably on a practice that allows either the quality of patient care to suffer or an overspend to happen. The basis of understanding the indicative budget is good sound financial control. In the past, the management accountant, who would have a better understanding of setting and monitoring budgets, undertook this role. This is slightly different to the role of the financial accountant, who would be more involved in actual costs.

Table 6: Key areas for maintaining good management

- The total value being managed (the indicative budget must be clearly understood)
- Have a robust plan in place that clearly identifies key monitoring criteria
- Adequate provision to support the process by employing appropriate staff rather than relying on existing personnel resources
- Regular management information should be readily available
- SLAs should be adhered to by both sides, i.e. commissioner and provider
- A feasible risk strategy, shared by both parties, should be in place
- Clear lines of communication should be established with all stakeholders, including the practice patients.

The above may seem obvious, but there are other issues that should be considered before undertaking the task of managing the indicative budget. Let us consider what may be actually happening during this control cycle.

The management cycle

It is likely that there will not be a clean sheet starting point. It is likely that where PCOs are experiencing brought-forward overspends, they will almost certainly address these deficits prior to releasing savings into primary care. This could mean that there is an additional element to be included into the commissioning plan.

The indicative budget should be clearly split into its component parts; this way all patient needs can be addressed. It is likely that there will not be enough money to cover every need. This is why there have always been waiting lists. The minimum and maximum waiting time should be clearly stated in the service level agreement.

What about exceptions? These will occur; typical events might include extra contractual referrals, either with or without prior approval. Another might be caused by a self-referral or overseas patients. Also, there is the issue of transient or temporary patients or expensive patients.

Overspends can and almost certainly will occur. Even the most robust plan can be affected by various factors. There can be a sudden increase in the number of patients caused by temporary or permanent factors. It is not possible to predict that every patient will be at the average cost. Complications and serious illness can lead to the high cost of expensive patients.

An understanding of inflationary costs should be included within the plan. If a private or alternative provider is used, then they may not necessarily maintain their prices at the same level throughout the whole year.

The first indicative budget should be underwritten by accurate data. Remember:

price of procedure x number of procedures = cost

Increased or reduced activity will result in an overspend or under-spend, respectively. Be aware of factors that could impact other services, such as increased or decreased waiting times, new procedures, or new medications and treatments.

The impact of patient choice

Notwithstanding all of the above, there is yet one more crucial factor that could very easily fragment even the most robust of financial plans. How do you deal with patient choice? In principle, payments by results should mean an equal playing field, but it is already clear that not all PCOs are progressing at the same rate. Key to this element is a clear understanding between the practice and PCT about how risk will be managed between both sides. List size variations and expensive patients are probably one of the highest risk areas and the practice needs to ensure that there is a locally agreed insurance plan. Some PCOs have agreed incentive schemes which sign the practice up to achieving quality indicators.

Having agreed how the indicative budget will be spent, it is important that the monitoring arrangements are suitable to ensure that the risk of overspending is kept to a minimum. Firstly, you must be able to define the level of activity; this is not just about recording what has taken place, but also being able to sensibly predict the level of future activity. Included within this activity might be certain quality measures, such as improved waiting times or more accessibility to services locally. The future financial commitment should be monitored regularly to avoid a drastic reduction of services towards the end of the financial year. For example, if more than 25% of the total resources have been committed by the end of the second month, then if everything remains equal, the allocation will have been fully used by the end of month eight, only two thirds through the financial year.

When agreeing the service level agreement, it is important that the key contract monitoring tools are identified. Typical indicators might include the following:

- Output data, e.g. definition of what constitutes an episode of care

- What is included in the cost and what is not, i.e. is the episode:

  - An outpatient appointment?
  - A day case?
  - A full consultant episode?
  - If the patient is admitted, what cost is going to be charged?

The least likely area to be developed at the moment surrounds quality indicators. However, there is a quick and easy way to review the service and that is by engaging in discussion with the practice patients. Each year the practice already carries out a survey, which could be expanded to cover commissioned services as well. The practice should not forget that there is a national service framework for core services already in place and it should look for evidence of this within the service being commissioned. The framework will cover the following key areas:

- The emphasis placed on improving health

- Services accessible to all

- Care delivered in an appropriate manner

- Services reflecting value for money

- Recording patient experience, i.e. the actual user of the service

- All health outcomes documented.

Payment terms

The commissioning cycle is to be governed by payment by results. This simply means that whoever actually carries out the work gets paid for it. What is therefore important from a management point of view is an absolutely clear definition about the terms for payment. For example, when will the invoice be issued and what method will the practice use to ensure that the activity has been carried out? Those involved in the commissioning during the days of fundholding will recall minimum data sets, i.e. the minimum data that will be accepted in quantifying and approving payments. This is vital when considering using the services of external providers. The practice should ensure that it can verify all activity with its own records. In the future, software may be introduced that can be accepted globally, but until such solutions exist it is important that the practice adopts its own method of data collection.

Both the practice and the provider will monitor their own initial data. The PCT will be responsible for monitoring both sets of data. The processes adopted will ensure that monitoring reports can be reviewed and, where deemed appropriate, quality audit visits can be arranged. Questionnaires and surveys can be utilised or new ones developed to assist in outcomes measurement. Communication needs to be maintained between all stakeholders via regular performance meetings.

Monitoring

Whilst the actual financial monitoring should be relatively straightforward, this will be based on actual data. Wherever there is a variance, this should be monitored in conjunction with the level of variance. As a priority, those areas where there is a greater variance should be investigated first. The financial variance is the easy part. Actually identifying why such a variance has occurred is not necessarily going to be straightforward and will involve discussion between stakeholders. This is probably the most interesting part of commissioning, because the causes for variations will not just be about financial variations, but will also involve clinical decisions about how care is delivered. The results of this monitoring will then inform the next commissioning cycle.

It is likely that whilst robust monitoring systems are developed there may be disputes between commissioner and provider. The PCT will act as an arbitration service and aim to resolve disputes locally. Where disputes cannot be resolved locally, they will be passed to the local strategic health authority, who will determine the dispute in favour of one of the parties. It is likely that the only disputes to be referred to this level will be those concerning the use of savings or where it has been decided that an indicative budget is to be removed.

The strategic health authority will report on an annual basis and review their findings regarding the operation of practice based commissioning in their own region.

Clinical audit

The Administrator will provide data for clinical audit and will probably be involved in the organisation of these data. They could participate in the planning of audits and make decisions on priorities.

The Manager will identify the clinical governance lead and could coordinate the same, and will be responsible for informing key staff about the outcomes of audits. They will also be responsible for the overall review of audits.

The Strategist will look at the complete cycle of clinical audits and where appropriate prioritise those areas that need most attention or improvement. For example, to achieve holistic points, it is necessary to achieve quality across a broad range of clinical domains. If too much effort is being expended in one area, the target maximum might be exceeded which, although positive in respect of quality in that particular area, might detract from other areas. Where a target maximum is exceeded, it will not generate additional points and receive no more financial incentive. Conversely, where targets are not achieved, the points obtained will be less than those available and will affect the financial incentive achieved. The same principle is applicable to commissioning secondary care services.

For information: *Each month identify the weakest area of the clinical audit (in respect of the clinical domain) and consider an action plan to make improvements.*

> **Advice tip:** When you have identified an area of weakness and have taken action to address it, make sure that you review the area again in a reasonable time (say 14 days) to ensure that changes are being made.

Organisational audit

The Administrator will provide and organise data to assist in the planning and understanding of processes within the practice.

The Manager will, under the direction of the GP, coordinate this information and also be responsible for ensuring the completion of the audit cycle.

The Strategist will not only comply and test the processes put in place, but could also be responsible for the development of existing, and introduction of new, procedures.

For information: *When evaluating processes, use simple models, such as a PDSA cycle. By using a method like this, you will be constantly reviewing and auditing your organisational structure.*

> **Advice tip:** If you evaluate processes correctly, you will realise that one PDSA cycle can lead to another or, in some cases, many other cycles. Remember this is a continuous programme of review.

Clinical effectiveness and evidence-based practice

The **Administrator** need not have an in-depth knowledge of this subject, but should be familiar with any issues and certainly have an understanding of the terminology used.

The **Manager** will need to have some knowledge of the local clinical effectiveness plans. This can be done by requesting information on priorities from the PCO. They will then be responsible for collecting data to measure these areas. As a result of this input, they might also be asked to assist in developing the practice's clinical effectiveness plan.

The **Strategist** will ensure that systems are in place to evaluate clinical effectiveness areas identified by the PCO and within the practice. They will also assist in identifying evidence-based practices; however, the latter should only be undertaken with input from the GP.

For information: *The practice will be demonstrating some of the above within the existing quality and outcomes framework. Therefore, keep the subject manageable; only pick one or two areas to concentrate on and link it to, say, existing work within the practice, such as a specialist clinic.*

> **Advice tip:** If the practice runs a clinic or service not carried out by others, then champion this and use its success to illustrate the commitment generally of the practice to providing quality services.

Service performance indicators

The **Administrator** should understand the terminology relating to specific service performance indicators. They will be able to collect data on key areas.

The **Manager** will use the above information and discuss practice performance with the lead GP against national and local performance standards.

The Strategist will mainly provide the necessary skills to analyse and evaluate how service indicators can be achieved. They should be able to identify the best systems to produce relevant results.

For information: *Define a specific list of performance indicators and use these in conjunction with those identified in the QOF.*

> **Advice tip:** You know your practice best; pick an area that you know well and use this as a personal measure of performance. For example, if you run a clinic that is a drop-in for patients other than your own, collate this data to demonstrate the usefulness of your specific service.

Service prioritisation

The Administrator will again collect data and assist the manager in service prioritisation issues.

The Manager will review the financial and human resources needed to support the identified services. They can deal directly with the PCO on new needs or revised priorities.

The Strategist will review services on a regular basis and establish the effectiveness of them. They will recommend changes where needed and ensure compliance to national and local targets. They should understand the commissioning process and be able to liaise with the PCO on commissioning issues that directly affect the practice.

For information: *Produce a list of the current service priorities and review these at least on an annual basis and amend as appropriate.*

> **Advice tip:** Very often the practice will apply for new resources to run its services and not receive anything. Keep this information alive so that it is possible to build up a stronger business case when new resources are identified. Remember, in the future it is to be payment by results.

The Effective Manager

1. Act on information, when it becomes available. Produce regular reports and act on outcomes when they are known. Look at the variances and try to make sure that you understand why such variances have occurred. Remember, you might have one area that is generating efficiencies, but no overall savings are made because another area is causing the indicative budget to overspend.

2. Plan ahead. Start to outline the practice intentions for the first three years. Create a rolling plan that can be adjusted to circumstances year on year.

3. Ensure any savings are invested wisely. Make sure that any investment into the practice brings longer-term benefits to the practice.

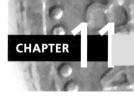
Budget setting methodology

The budget setting methodology will be slightly different in each region or locality, because local issues and the speed of introduction will be determined by the readiness of both the practices and providers to engage in a full commissioning model.

The budget setting methodology will break the indicative budget down into key areas. These areas could include the following:

- Planned inpatient activity

- Planned day case activity

- Outpatient (first appointment)

- Outpatient (follow-ups)

- Emergency admissions

- Walk in A&E admissions

- Regular attenders

- Enhanced services

- PMS, GMS, alternative PMS

- Private providers

- Diagnostics

- Prescribing

- GP urgent referrals

The above list is not necessarily exhaustive and may include more or less in each local area.

The key principles

The key principles of the budget setting methodology are based upon local agreement and voluntary participation by the practice. However, even if the practice is not actively involved in the commissioning process, it can still ask to receive an indicative budget; this budget will cover all areas of patient care. It is unlikely that this approach will be needed; however, the practice should be aware that this right does exist in case local negotiations, in the form of consortium arrangements, do not suit completely the aims of the practice. In most cases, development is being undertaken to put in place local consortium arrangements covering a group of patients in locally defined areas. The resulting budget agreed will be referred to as the default budget and will develop into a genuine local budget over a period of time.

If an area already has good data, there is nothing to stop them using it to inform the budget setting process. For example, work has been undertaken on identifying clinical pathways *(see Appendix A)*, which has already helped the decision making process, determining where services should be commissioned.

A default budget

During the financial year 2005/06, the aim is to create a default budget that covers elective inpatient and day case activity only. This does not mean that where local methods have been established they cannot be used during 2005/06. The main reason for this (with the exception of those trusts that have achieved foundation status) is that for inpatient and day case activity the national tariff will apply. All other services will be agreed locally, which is why there will be a variation of how services are costed, area-by-area. This means that there can be a discrepancy of prices across health authority or PCT boundaries. This could be quite important when considering the patient choice agenda in respect of providers offered to patients.

Local arrangements will expect to cover a full range of services, but it must be stressed that the final budget allocation will be derived from two distinct methods of calculating the indicative budget. There are also likely to be exceptions made. The PCT will need to monitor local arrangements to ensure that there is no inappropriate transfer of activity or significant change to referral patterns.

Hospital Episode Statistics (HES), which have been evaluated for 2003/04 will be used to form the basis of the budget for most practices. This data will be made available to PCTs when it has been collated, broken down to practice level. When the PCT receive it, they will be free to aggregate the data into groups of practices, where local consortium arrangements have been agreed.

The importance of local factors

Remember that, ultimately, the level of initial budgets set will be partially determined by local factors. In particular, where a PCT is already overspent it can take this into consideration when agreeing local budgets. Therefore it may not be unusual, in the first couple of years of commissioning, that efficiency savings will be allocated against such overspends in the first instance. The budget will take into account local historical activity, the tariff price and the PCT's current financial position. The final size of the allocated budget will also be determined by the locally agreed strategy for risk management.

So, to summarise, the 2005/06 budget will be based on 2003/04 historical data, which will be adjusted for increased activity (patient demand) and changes to list sizes. Where clinical pathways have changed or services have already been moved from secondary care to primary care, this will also be taken into account.

This method of setting the budget means that the use of historical data may actually initially reward those practices that have been high referrers, and funds will not necessarily be distributed based on true need. However, by 2006/07, it will be expected that the basis of budget distribution will be equalised between practices, irrespective of historical referral patterns.

The core data for 2003/04 should be updated for inflation for 2004/05 and 2005/06; the exception to this will be areas covered by payment by results, which will be carried by the published tariff. Local delivery plans will form the basis of how monies will be distributed and form the basis for discussion to benchmark activity and cost. However, PCTs will still have the flexibility to select their own information regarding activity growth, and not necessarily use the average data provided by the SHA.

One area that may affect the indicative budget is the possibility of list size changes. It is important that consideration is given to list size changes from 2003/04 through to 2005/06.

The basic concept

Firstly, identify the practice list size as at April 2003 and April 2004, and break down the list by the following age range:

0-4   5-14   15-44   45-64   65-74   75-84   85+

Once the lists have been defined, an average list is created by age, by adding the two lists together and dividing by two. This will give rise to average weighted list size for the practice. The average list is then calculated by applying the following cost weightings:

0-4	5-14	15-44	45-64	65-74	75-84	85+
542.04	269.01	525.78	655.41	1245.37	1976.50	2799.20

During the first quarter of 2005, the population breakdown should be identified, and the age cost weighted list for 2005 can then be calculated. Now the 2003/04 average costed list can be compared with 2005 and this will give rise to an uplift or decrease of the 2003/04 budget.

Sounds simple? In all the years that I have been involved in general practice, there have always been discussions about list sizes and why they may not be accurate at any given time. Ghost patients, transient populations, temporary residents, changes in social circumstances and housing policies, can all contribute to why sometimes list sizes cannot be verified or agreed. Whenever list sizes form part of the budget setting methodology, it leads to a measurable way of either increasing or decreasing budgets.

Payment by results

In 2002, it was agreed that there would be the largest increase in NHS funding over a five-year period. This would average 7.4% real growth per year, with the intention of matching the European average by the year 2008.

It is now 2006 and with the introduction of the new contract, we are seeing contract values increasing by 3.225%, in addition to requests for referral rates to be cut by 3.25% to offset brought-forward secondary care deficits. So are the new resources being used effectively and demonstrating good value for money? If the introduction of practice based commissioning so far is anything to go by, it may not at first glance appear to be achieving its aims.

A good thing about the new financial system means that there will be, in theory, a documented audit trail about how money is being allocated. However, consider the two models below:

Historic Budget #1	**Historic Budget #2**
Fully costed at historic levels	Fully costed at historic levels, less 10% contingency fund (for risk management)

Both models will be expected to stay within budget; which model would you prefer? Anyway, let us consider the reality - the new financial model will need to deliver the following:

1. Reward genuine efficiency

2. Support patient choice

3. Allow diversity and case mix

4. Generate waiting time reductions.

There are two real key factors to the process. The provider will be paid for the actual activity that they undertake. They will be paid at an agreed tariff price; this will be the national tariff, but even in these cases the price may be varied to take into account local cost pressures on price variation, such as wages and living costs.

What has been happening for 2005/06?

The financial model is meant to address the requirement to create a more personalised service for patients. This is designed to be delivered over a ten-year time span. As stated before, there is to be an average increase of 7.4% a year over and above inflation. This is represented by an increase of 45% (£34 billion) from 2003/04 to 2007/08; this represents a change from £56 billion in 2003/04 to £90 billion by 2007/08. Given all this funding, the model is expected to deliver effective services that are responsive to patient needs. It is expected to allow the development of a greater range of service providers and becomes a robust financial model that will sustain the above. Foundation Trusts have been involved in payment by results since April 2004 and by 2005 all trusts had become involved in some shape or form.

The price that is set needs to be fair to both the provider and the commissioner. However, the aim of this system is eventually to have a set of tariff prices that are applicable whenever or wherever the activity is actually carried out.

What will the tariff cover? Ultimately ALL activity will be covered by the tariff. This will include:

- Inpatient
- Day case
- Outpatient
- A&E
- Mental health
- Community services
- Some primary care

The above is not exhaustive, but is illustrative of the key elements. Because of limited data and other information, it is envisaged that for 2005/06 and maybe 2006/07, that this will be limited to only the following:

- Outpatients
- Critical care episodes
- A&E
- Possibly mental health and community health services

Due to the transition of various models and local interpretation, it has been decided that the financial model will be established over a three-year period from 2005/06 to 2007/08.

Table 7: The three-year financial model

Year One (05/06)

The PCT will effectively maintain a status quo retaining their full purchasing power, but will start working practices to establish the first tranche of indicative budgets.

Years Two and Three (06/07) and (07/08)

A move to tariff prices is made creating a maximum efficiency saving of 9% over three years.

The Effective Manager

1. In 2005/06, understand the basic concept of practice based commissioning

2. By 2006/07, be actively involved in commissioning processes in your practice

3. By 2007/08, be fully conversant with practice based commissioning and make it work for your patients and the practice.

Appendix A: Care pathways

As part of the new contract, the practice manager should possess certain core competencies of which care pathways are one. The following illustrates the level of expertise expected of the practice:

The Administrator must be able to demonstrate an understanding of care pathways and will be able to participate in pathway mapping and design. Very often the administrator knows the staff attached to the practice and the services they provide, but often it is not clearly documented who does what or when.

The Manager will take responsibility for coordinating the above and ensuring that it is implemented and reviewed when appropriate. Very often a community midwife will attend the surgery at the same time each week, but in fact this might not make best use of existing practice space or resources. By discussion and evaluation of the need, a change of date, or time, or even location will actually improve the service.

The Strategist will ensure the smooth implementation and review of care pathways. They will also be responsible for evaluating the effectiveness and making changes where necessary. They should be able to advise the practice on the principles, which are chiefly to provide a tool and a concept that demonstrate clear guidelines and protocols. These should be locally agreed, evidence-based, but more importantly, patient-centered. The Strategist will be able to ensure that for the practice, the right people are doing the right things in the correct order at the right time in the right place with the correct or desired outcome. All of this will be done with consideration of the practice population needs; there is no point in developing care pathways that do not reflect the requirements of the practice patient population.

Evaluate the services available and amend them according to demand and effectiveness.

Appendix B: Risk management

Risk management can be defined in numerous ways and covers various areas within the practice. This appendix will cover each area from the obvious risks posed to staff and patients in a busy working environment, to the less obvious risks associated with planning services. Risk can be preventative, but can also be rewarding. Whatever the purpose for assessing the risk, it is important to understand how the assessment can be judged to ensure the right outcome for the practice.

The obvious risk associated with practice based commissioning is that of ensuring that there are sufficient incentives given to practices to encourage active participation, but at the same time not too much to undermine the very infrastructure of delivering high quality care. The introduction of payment by results means that a clear understanding of commissioning strategies at PCT, locality and practice level must be defined. For 2005/06 payment by results will be restricted to certain elective activities and therefore the risk for the PCT will be lower than in future years. Now is the time to consider alternatives to hospital episodes, so that the risk factors can be better managed from 2006/07.

There is no specific risk management strategy that should be adopted, but advice has been put forward that suggests the following basic principles be adopted. The PCT may wish to top-slice the overall allocation, thereby creating a fixed sum for use as a contingency fund. If such a policy is adopted, it will be important that there are clearly defined parameters for calling on such contingency funds. In theory, the principle is fine, but it does lead to the debate that demands placed on the reserve fund could be looked upon as being short-term loans that demand future repayment. Indeed, persistent claims made against the reserve could lead to reduced budgets or even exclusion from holding a budget.

This fund could be treated as a recurring adjustment or a non-recurring adjustment, depending on local factors. Should the contingency fund not be completely exhausted at the end of the year, then the surplus would be released to practices to fund future service developments. The real problem with this approach is that it means that the practice will commence the year with a reduced budget; a budget that will not address the needs of the historical baseline. Where a PCT is already holding a deficit, the degree of risk is heightened. A cynical view would be that practice based commissioning is about using practice resources to resolve such deficits on behalf of the PCT. To establish a robust risk management strategy, it is key to the process that local variations or policies are fully understood.

Appendix C: Choose and book

As from now, patients who require any form of elective treatment will be offered a choice of appointment and at least an opportunity to choose from four providers once their GP has decided that a referral is necessary.

Choose and book is to be a nationally recognised service to patients that will combine electronic booking and a choice of time, date and place for the first outpatient appointment. It is in principle the same concept of booking an airline ticket at the travel agent or using the internet. It is envisaged that it will be available to all patients in England requiring elective care. This represents over 10 million patients per year. Patients needing elective treatment will be offered a choice of at least four providers and in some cases even more, once their GP has decided that a referral is actually necessary and appropriate. These providers could be NHS trusts, foundation trusts, treatment centres, private hospitals or practitioners with a special interest operating within primary care.

In the future it is possible that alternative types of providers will emerge as a result of practice based commissioning. The practice has a real opportunity to influence change in this area. As well as choosing where they go, patients will be able to choose when they go by phoning an appointments line, booking over the internet, or booking at the GP surgery. This all sounds fine, but the reality will be a potential nightmare if choice is exercised completely. The system assumes a fair share concept, but it will be inevitable that certain providers will be favoured over others. To combat the problem of different lengths of waiting times, the current idea is for any patient who has to wait longer than six months for an operation to be offered a choice of an alternative place of treatment. This is called 'choice at six months'.

Appendix D: Patient choice and patient choice at six months

Patient choice is due to be introduced to the NHS from January 2006. However, it was meant to be introduced in 2005 and currently not all practices are geared up for this initiative. Linked to this is 'patient choice at six months', which is largely untested and relies on patient choice working in the first place. The following explains the principles of patient choice and patient choice at six months.

Patient choice, or at least the concept that it implies, is probably the single most determining factor when implementing the concept of practice based commissioning. This is because practice based commissioning is designed to engage patients in the decision making process about how future services will be commissioned. At the same time, patients will be advised that they may elect to choose their service provider at the time of booking the appointment. This means that these providers will need to be within the commissioning framework. As more and more services are included and patients start to engage in the process, then more and more services will be defined by actual patient choice. This will of course take time to evolve, but it will be interesting to see how existing providers react to these real decisions. It will also be interesting to see what new innovations appear and how new providers will offer services.

Since the middle of 2004, patients who have had to wait more than six months for elective surgery have been offered the choice of moving to another hospital for quicker treatment. Patients will be notified about their choice options. Conversely, patients may still continue to choose to wait for an appointment at their chosen hospital if they wish. Patients who are expected to wait more than six months will be contacted at the earliest opportunity and certainly before they have waited five months. Patients may need to be contacted earlier to allow an offer of faster treatment. However, what is not made clear here is that the waiting time is calculated from the point that the first appointment is acknowledged. Therefore, it does not take account of the time that has elapsed from the point of the initial referral. If the scheme is to work, then waiting times will become more precisely measured, i.e. when the patient is given the flexibility to book the appointments directly.

The alternative that will be offered to the patient will guarantee that the treatment will take place and could include the use of private treatment centres. The patient will be offered a confirmed pre-booked appointment. Of course, although the patient will have waited more than six months to qualify for this option, it may still be possible that they might not be seen for another three months. Transport will be provided to patients who otherwise would not be able to attend the offered facility.

Appendix E: Foundation Trusts

The Health and Social Care Act 2003 established NHS Foundation Trusts as independent public benefit corporations.

- They are under local control, utilising local public accountability rather than central controls

- The foundation trust will be entitled to retain any surpluses and look at new ways of raising capital for investing in new services

- They will have complete control in the recruitment and employment of their own staff

- They will need to deliver against national targets and general standards as per all other parts of the NHS; however, they will be free to decide how they achieve this

- They will not be restricted by directions from the Secretary of State for Health

- They will not be subject to the same performance management criteria as set by strategic health authorities or the Department of Health.

NHS Foundation Trusts form part of a major programme of investment, expansion and reform of the NHS over a ten year period. The concept of Foundation will benefit both patients and Trust staff. Freedom to innovate will improve services to patients continuing to meet the service needs of patients irrespective of their ability to pay.

The success or failure of Foundation Trusts will have implications on how practice based commissoiing is percieved. Bear in mind that Foundation Trusts will develop services without the interference from central government. It will be interesting to see how they plan to develop services in conjunction with local practice based commissioning agendas.

Appendix F: PCT checklist for practice based commissioning

This is a broad framework that gives an indication of the processes that the PCT is likely to follow to ensure that it implements practice based commissioning in the most sensitive and fair way. The good manager will need to understand the processes that the PCT adopts because its approach will have a direct impact on any additional work being undertaken at practice level.

Y/N	PCT checklist for practice based commissioning
	PCT/Practice Relationships
☐	Has the practice/group demonstrated collaborative working?
☐	Is there sufficient clinical engagement?
☐	Have natural commissioning units been identified?
	Practice Competency
☐	Has the practice demonstrated levels of commissioning competency?
☐	Has the practice demonstrated levels of management competency?
☐	PCT competency?
☐	Have staff resources been identified?
	Aims and Objectives
☐	Are aims/objectives clear?
☐	Are outcomes clear?

Y/N	PCT checklist for practice based commissioning
☐	Have key services been identified?
☐	Have service level agreements for PBC been identified?
☐	Has the scale/scope of implementation been planned?

Finance

☐	Are budgets clearly identified?
☐	Has the process for moving to weighted capitation budgets been agreed?

Clinical Governance

☐	Is the accountability framework clear?
☐	Have local PBC quality standards been agreed?
☐	Have monitoring arrangements been established?
☐	Is the practice/PCT shared agreement in place?
☐	Can patient choice assurances be given?
☐	Are key roles identified?
☐	Is the decision-making mechanism clear?

IT and Data

☐	Have possible IT solutions been explored?
☐	Has the identification and feedback of key practice data been established?
☐	Is the process for using quality data clear?

Y/N	PCT checklist for practice based commissioning
☐	Are support personnel identified and trained?
☐	Does the PCT have the resources to develop monitoring tools as necessary?
	PCT Management
☐	Is the PCT leadership clear?
	Communication
☐	Have practices been informed of the local delivery plan?
☐	Has the PCT informed practices of key PBC focus areas and plans for implementation and support?
☐	Has communication with key stakeholders been established?
☐	Has internal communication in PCT been undertaken?
	Evaluation and review of local PBC
☐	Has the PCT put in place a process for evaluating local PBC implementation?
☐	Has the PCT put in place a process for monitoring the impact of PBC?

Appendix G: Practice checklist for practice based commissioning

Practices that take part in practice based commissioning will be expected to make a formal application to participate to their responsible PCT. The following checklist will provide the basic information to inform the practice and the PCT of whether the practice is ready to undertake commissioning. It forms the basis of any local application by a practice or group of practices to join the scheme.

Y/N	Practice checklist for practice based commissioning

1. Strategy

☐ Can the practice satisfy key local aims and objectives of PBC as defined?*

☐ Has the practice addressed issues locally and the local delivery plan?*

☐ Has the practice demonstrated how key outcomes can be delivered?*

* In each of the above the practice will list two or three key objectives

2. Accountability

☐ Does the practice/PCT have a shared agreement in place?

☐ Is there a locality agreement in place?

☐ Are the practice leadership and management structures clear?

☐ Is the practice management capacity clear and sustainable?

☐ Does the practice offer choice?

Y/N	Practice checklist for practice based commissioning

3. Financial

☐ Has the practice identified the level of management cost required?

☐ Has the level of potential overall savings been assessed?

☐ Has the practice ensured financial risks to the practice/locality have been assessed?

☐ Is the practice confident that this level of service/funding can be sustained?

☐ Are the practice priorities for re-investment stated?

☐ Is IT in place or has data validation taken place?

4. Service provision

☐ Does the application maintain local stability of services and equity across practices and locality?

☐ Has the practice made an assessment of current services?

☐ Has the number of patients benefiting been determined?

☐ Is the practice satisfied with the balance between the number of patients benefiting compared to the whole PCT population?

☐ Would the practice be happy with the possibility of roll out to a wider PCT area if successful?

5. Proposed timetable (new arrangements proposed start date):

☐ 2005/6

☐ 2006/7

☐ 2007/8

Y/N	Practice checklist for practice based commissioning

6. Key stakeholders and patient involvement

☐ Can the involvement of patients be substantiated?

☐ Are community groups involved?

7. Practice representatives

☐ Have key leads at the practice been identified?

☐ Has the practice provided contact details?

Appendix H: Sample Service Level Agreement

The attached is just an example, but gives a flavour of what you might expect to see in the practice service level agreement:

SERVICE LEVEL AGREEMENT BETWEEN

"The Commissioner": *enter Practice Name or Group Name (list all partners)*

and

"The Provider": *Example – ABC Hospital Trust*

A. SERVICE LEVEL AGREEMENT   SUMMARY SHEET

Name of Service(s):

Service Provider Contact:

Service Provider Address:

Telephone No. Email:

Fax:

Commissioning Contact:

Commissioning Address:

Telephone No./Email:

Fax:

Agreement Period:

Start Date:

End Date:

Review Dates:

Payment Arrangements:

Overall Value of SLA:

Signed for and on behalf of Commissioner:

Name:

Designation:

Signature:

Signed for and on behalf of Service Provider:

Name:

Designation:

Signature:

Reference No.

Complaints

Confidentiality

Data Protection Act Compliance

Insurance

Access to Records

Staff

Asylum and Immigration Act Compliance

Management Arrangements

Quality Assurance System

Quality Control

Monitoring

Entitlement to Contract

Assignments and Under-letting of Agreement

Cancellation of SLA in case of improper practice, etc.

Definition of Force Majeure

Termination of Agreement

Disputes and arbitration

B. SERVICE AGREEMENT SPECIFICATION(S)

B.1: Name of Service

B.2: Strategic Objectives

B.3: Funding Breakdown/Budget Breakdown

B.4: Objectives of Service

B.5: Description of Service

B.6: (a) Target Group(s)/Criteria for Service
(b) Review Process for Eligible Need

B.7: Catchment Area of Service

B.8: Outcome/Target Measurement

B.9: User Consultation

Reference No.

C. SERVICE AGREEMENT CONDITIONS

C.1: Agreement Type

Fixed Term – 1 year

Fixed Term – 3 year

3 year rolling, subject to annual review

Select the type of contract term as appropriate

C.2: Funding Arrangements

Where upon receipt of the statistical information required under Clause D1 and D2 it appears that the service targets have not been achieved, the commissioner may deduct from the next or any subsequent payment to be made, a sum which represents a fair and reasonable amount in respect of the shortfall in the service targets.

C.3: Mutual Responsibilities

Commissioner:
To provide support when required through the commissioning contact
To issue payments, as agreed
To monitor service provided
To work in the formulation of policy and service developments
To ensure a quality, value for money service
To keep informed of the likely funding in respect of the next financial year
Unless otherwise notified, the above responsibilities will be undertaken by the commissioner

Service Provider:

To provide the services specified in this agreement

To provide statistical information to the commissioner as detailed

To inform the commissioner of any problems which may result in failure of the service or part thereof

To keep the commissioner informed of all developments or changes in plans for the service

To work with and support target group(s) as stated

To keep up to date with appropriate legislation

C.4: Health and Safety

The provider shall operate and update a Health and Safety Policy compliant with the Health and Safety at Work Act 1974, Section 2(3) which places duty upon both Employers and Employees.

C.5: Equal Opportunities

In delivering the service, the provider will not discriminate against any individual on the grounds of race, sex, colour, religious beliefs, disability or any other circumstances listed in the commissioner's Equal Opportunities Policy.

C.6: Access to Services

The provider will comply with the Disability Discrimination Act and all related legislation and have regard to any relevant Government Codes of Practice and Guidance.

C.7: Complaints

The provider will set out clear procedures for dealing with clients' complaints. These procedures must include a written record of all client complaints and any action taken. This record to be available for inspection by the commissioner.

C.8: Confidentiality

Neither party shall use or disclose any information concerning the business or other affairs of the other party, or any information concerning the affairs of any service user save for:

- Information in the public domain (other than by breach of this clause)

- Information which the recipient is obliged to disclose by law.

C.9: Data Protection Act Compliance

The provider shall at all times for the duration of the contract, comply with the requirements of the Data Protection Act 1998 and in particular, without prejudice to the generality of the foregoing shall have appropriate technical and organisational security measures in place to prevent unauthorised or unlawful processing of personal information, and to prevent accidental loss, destruction or damage to any personal information they hold or process.

C.10: Insurance

The provider will be required to arrange and maintain a level of insurance which complies with current statutory requirements. The provider will produce evidence of insurance for inspection upon demand if required by the commissioner.

C.11: Access to Records

The commissioner's designated representative has the right to inspect all records of the provider relating to the agreement and/or service and have the right to interview all of the provider's staff who have been involved, either directly or indirectly, with the conduct or administration of the agreement.

C.12: Staff

The appointment of staff, including volunteers, should be subject to the organisation's own risk assessment process and include the provision of two satisfactory written references, one of which should be from a previous employer (where applicable). These should be obtained before individuals commence employment. The provider's recruitment process should ensure that all staff and volunteers who work on a one to-one basis with vulnerable people and children are subject to appropriate checks. Other staff and volunteers will be subject to checks at the discretion of, and be the responsibility of, the provider. Staff employed for the service shall be suitably qualified and trained to meet the needs of the patients.

C.13: Asylum and Immigration Act Compliance

The provider is advised that their recruitment processes should include checking the right to work through compliance with the Asylum and Immigration Act 1998 without discriminating unlawfully.

C.14: Management Arrangements

The provider will send the commissioner an organisational chart detailing the staffing and management arrangements for the service.

C.15: Quality Assurance System

The provider will have in operation certain quality systems as agreed with the commissioner.

C.16: Quality Control

The provider will have in operation a quality control system consistent with standards approved by the commissioner, which will include inspection of service detail and measures for improvement. Service inspection and monitoring procedures should be tailored to meet the needs of the service.

C.17: Monitoring

The commissioner or designated representatives reserve the right to visit the provider with or without notice. The commissioner reserves the right to audit source data relating to the services provided. The provider shall make all relevant records available for inspection upon receiving reasonable notice (anonymised where necessary).

C.18: Entitlement to Contract

This is not an exclusive agreement and the commissioner reserves the right to contract with any other alternative provider, other than the provider, for the supply and delivery of similar services.

C.19: Assignments and Under-letting of Agreement

The provider shall not assign or under-let the agreement or any part of it and shall not sub-contract except with the written consent of the commissioner.

C.20: Cancellation of SLA in case of improper practice, etc

The PCT shall be empowered to cancel the agreement if the provider is guilty of any improper or corrupt practice.

C.21: Force Majeure

The provider shall not be liable for default arising from circumstances beyond its reasonable control (such as, but not restricted to, flood, fire and civil unrest), but the PCT shall in such circumstances be entitled to take such action as is deemed necessary to protect the interests of the patients and make a fair and reasonable adjustment to the price.

C.22: Termination of Agreement

Where either party is in breach of the provisions of this agreement and that breach is capable of remedy, the other party may serve notice upon the party in breach, specifying the breach complained of and requiring rectification of that breach within 28 days. If the breach is not remedied in accordance with such notice, the party serving the notice may terminate the agreement forthwith by notice in writing. Where either party is in breach of the provisions of the agreement and that breach is not capable of remedy, the other party may terminate the agreement forthwith by giving written notice to the party in breach. This agreement may in any case be terminated by either party giving the other not less than three to six months prior notice in writing at any time, subject to individual circumstances.

C.23: Disputes

The parties to the contract will use their best endeavours to resolve by negotiation any dispute arising out of or relating to the agreement. Where resolution is not agreed between the parties, conciliation by an independent person, agreed between the parties may be sought who shall recommend the terms of the settlement.

D. MONITORING ARRANGEMENTS (SUMMARY)

The following information will be made available to the commissioner by the provider.

D.1: Statistical Information

State frequency

D.2: Qualitative Information

State frequency

E. SERVICE LEVEL AGREEMENT CODE OF BEST PRACTICE

A Code of Best Practice has been developed to identify the basis of Service Level Agreements between practices and providers. Any defined local code of best practice will be included here.

F. MONITORING TEMPLATE

Date of monitoring visit: ....

Constitution on file Y/N

Up-to-date General Report/Financial Statement on file Y/N

F.1 Name of Provider: ....

SLA status - Nature of visit:

Work in progress

Awaiting hard copy

Complete

Date completed: ....

F.2 Present:

Name: .... Role:...

Name: .... Role:...

F.3 Funding:

Comments:...

....

....

F.4 Development of Service

Comments:...

....

....

F.5 Service Targets/Outcomes (see statistical information)

Targets/Outcomes evidenced:

Comments:...

....

....

F.6 Stakeholder Consultation

Methods evidenced:

Comments:...

....

....

F.7 Insurance

Certificate evidenced : ....

Comments:...

....

....

F.8 Personnel/Recruitment Systems:

Evidenced Records of Best Practice:

	Staff / Volunteer	Sample 1	Sample 2	Sample 3
Job Description				
References				
CRB				
Qualifications				
Contract				
Induction				
Training				
Supervision				

Comments:...

....

....

Policies and Procedures of the Organisation (suggested list)

Mandatory (M) Contractual (C) Good Practice (G) Discretionary (D)

Status	Policy/Procedure	Evidenced	Comments
M/C	Health and Safety		
	- Moving and Handling (if applicable)		
	- Risk Assessment		
M/C	Fire Safety		
M/C	Adult Protection		
M/C	Data Protection		
M/C	Confidentiality		

C	Aims/Objectives – Mission Statement
C	Organisational Chart
C	Code of Practice - Standards
C	Constitution
G	Service User Guide
M/C	Equal Opportunities
G	Conflict of Interest
G	Handling Money
G	Recording of incidents affecting service users or their property
G	Liaison with linked professionals and/or carer relative of the service users
G	Key Holding Policy
G	Recording systems, e.g. service user information, provision record

Personnel Policies and Practices:

G	Recruitment and Selection
M/C	CRB – Declaration of offences
M/C	Asylum and Immigration Check
G	Job Descriptions
G	Contract of Employment
G	Induction Programme
G	Ongoing Staff Training
G	Staff Supervision/Appraisal Process
G	Disciplinary Procedure
G	Grievance Procedure

Quality Assurance:

C	Quality Assurance System, e.g. IIP, Internal
C	Complaints Procedure/Log

G	Marketing Information
C	Annual/Financial Reports
C	Quality Control System – Mechanism to check standards of service
C	Service User Consultation/Satisfaction
G	Whistle Blowing Policy

Agreed Action Plan	By whom	Date

Signed by: .... Manager:...

Commissioner's Representative: ....

G: SERVICE LEVEL AGREEMENT – GUIDANCE NOTES / GLOSSARY

Definition of the Service Level Agreement:

A Service Level Agreement is an agreement between two or more legal parties for the provision of services at an agreed level of quantity and quality. When the contract is with an NHS organisation, the Service Level Agreement is referred to as a 'Section 28a Transfer of Memorandum of agreement' for legal purposes.

Section A – Service Level Agreement Summary Sheet

1. **Name of Service:** This refers to the specific service. The service title(s) may differ from the provider's name, as there may be more than one service provided. Should this be the case, the services will be detailed individually and attached as a Schedule A.

2. **Commissioning Contact:** This is the identified person from the commissioning body taking the monitoring lead, e.g. PCT.

3. **Agreement Period:** This denotes the length of the contract.

4. **Review Dates:** This denotes the frequency of the review.

5. **Payment Arrangements:** This denotes the frequency of payment and may vary between commissioning bodies. When the commissioning body is an NHS organisation, the provider completes and returns the 'Section 28a annual voucher' to obtain payment (or locally agreed equivalent).

6. **Overall Value:** This is the total sum of all services listed that are covered by the Service Level Agreement.

Section B – Service Agreement Specification

1. **Name of Service:** There may be more than one service with different specifications. Should this be the case, the services will be detailed individually and attached as a Schedule A.

2. **Strategic Objectives:** This identifies the strategic objectives/targets that the service addresses in order to meet Government targets, e.g. NHS Plan, Community Plan, Local Delivery Plan.

3. **Funding Breakdown:** This denotes the breakdown of the contributions made. It may also include external sources of funding, if appropriate.

Budget Breakdown: This should be presented as capital and revenue costs for each year of the SLA. Capital costs are one-off costs such as materials and computer equipment. Revenue costs are ongoing yearly costs for the life of the SLA such as salaries, utilities or rent. This will be adjusted over time as we move towards a national tariff and payment by results.

Direct NHS Funded:

Include bank details for payment.

Include an auditor's certificate, which will be completed by the NHS auditor.

4. **Objectives of Service:** This denotes *what* the service is going to do, e.g. to provide a day case service.

Direct NHS Funded:

Briefly explain the benefits of providing the service external to NHS.

5. **Description of Service:** This denotes *how* the service will be provided, e.g. five days per week, 9am-5pm, etc.

6. **(a) Target Groups/Criteria for Service:** This identifies the key target groups and indicates eligible need, e.g. visual impairment, disabled, older people, age group, black & minority ethnic, diagnosis.

    (b) Review Process for Eligible Need: This refers to the process of checking that the service user still meets the criteria B6(a), e.g. formal, informal, frequency, recording.

7. **Catchment Area of Service:** This indicates the area that the service covers, e.g. patient catchment area.

8. **Outcome/Target Measurement:** This reflects the measurable number/output anticipated, e.g. 50-day case episodes, 40 elective inpatient appointments.

9. **User Consultation:** This reflects the method that service users are involved in for the development of the service, e.g. questionnaire, discussion groups, annual feedback.

Section C – Service Agreement Conditions

This section reflects a number of legal clauses that are required in a formal contract and that have been agreed by the commissioning unit's legal departments. Some clauses are not applicable to all providers.

1. **Agreement Type:** This denotes the status/term of the agreement.

2. **Funding Arrangements:** This refers to the possible financial consequences should the provider not fulfil their service targets. The commissioners may claw back a sum of money reflecting the shortfall.

Direct NHS Funded:

The audit statement should be completed by the NHS audit commission (REFER TO PCT FOR FULL DETAILS) in order to satisfy section 28a requirements.

3. **Mutual Responsibilities:** This denotes the duties placed upon the participants to the Service Level Agreement.

4. **Health and Safety:** For further information see: www.hse.gov.uk.

5. **Equal Opportunities:** For further information contact the local PCT.

6. **Access to Services:** For further information see: www.disability.gov.uk.

7. **Complaints:** For further information contact the local PCT.

8. **Confidentiality:** For further information contact the local PCT.

9. **Data Protection Act Compliance:** For further information see: www.hmso.gov.uk.

10. **Insurance:** Public Liability refers to third party property damage and bodily injury. The limit should be assessed against the possible worst-case scenario. For further information contact your insurance broker.

11. **Access to Records:** This allows access by the commissioners to inspect your financial records relating to the Service Level Agreement, with prior agreement.

12. **Staff:** For further information on recruitment contact the local PCT. For further information regarding Criminal Records Disclosure, see www.crb.gov.uk.

13. **Asylum and Immigration Act Compliance:** For further information see: www.hmso.gov.uk.

14. **Management Arrangements:** These are required to evidence adequate management of the service.

15. **Quality Assurance System:** A quality assurance system is a framework of

processes that ensure continuous improvement for the organisation. The system must include: equal opportunities, staff supervision/appraisal, record keeping, customer satisfaction, etc. Quality systems may be nationally recognised.

16. **Quality Control:** This is a framework of processes that allow checking/inspection of systems to ensure quality. This may include client/staff records, call-backs (telephones) and complaints. There may be circumstances which determine a visit without due notice.

17. **Monitoring:** Processes are in place to help raise standards and offer guidance and ensure that the contract is being met. This may be in addition to the formal review dates. See Section D for further information.

18. **Entitlement to Contract:** For further information contact the local PCT.

19. **Assignments and Under-letting of Agreement:** For further information contact the local PCT.

20. **Cancellation of SLA in Case of Improper Behaviour, etc:** For further information contact the local PCT.

21. **Force Majeure:** For further information contact the local PCT.

22. **Termination of Agreement:** For further information contact the local PCT.

23. **Disputes:** For further information contact the local PCT.

Section D – Monitoring Arrangements

1. **Statistical Information:** commissioners will require statistical evidence to be submitted on an agreed basis to demonstrate that the targets/outcomes. described in B.4 and B.8 are being met. These may be collected using the statistics form or other approved form.

2. **Qualitative Information:** commissioners will require reports to be submitted on an agreed basis to demonstrate the activities/developments of the service covered by the Service Level Agreement.

Section F – Monitoring Template

In order to meet Standing Orders and Audit requirements of the local PCT, regular monitoring of performance is carried out to ensure compliance with the Service Level Agreement. This function is measured against the agreed objectives of the funding and used to support future funding decisions. Service monitoring assists in identifying service gaps for future planning needs and promoting partnerships working towards the development of services. The contract monitoring procedure is a function that is devoted to continuous improvement and to raising standards, together with the ultimate aim of providing quality services for the benefit of service users.

1. **Name of Provider/SLA Status:** This is to identify the current situation with regards to the progress of the SLA.

2. **Present:** Lists all individuals at monitoring visit.

3. **Funding:** This will note any recent changes or anticipated requirements to be forwarded on to the budget holder.

4. **Development of Service:** This will document any service gaps and planned changes for the service.

5. **Service Targets/Outcomes:** This is evidenced in statistics forms (Appendix 3), which have been submitted prior to the meeting. Information gathered can be used as a planning tool for the future.

6. **User Consultation:** This is evidenced in reports, questionnaires, minutes and outcomes, etc. Consultation with service users is an important element to the planning/commissioning process.

7. **Insurance:** This will require evidence of certificates for insurance identified.

8. **Personnel/Recruitment Systems:** This is to evidence, by sample, the systems in place to support continuous improvement and quality. Any gaps in training needs and/or qualifications may be identified and arranged through working together with other agencies, ensuring continuous improvement in services.

9. **Policies and Procedures of the Organisation:** This is to evidence policies and procedures that are in place to ensure quality systems. Those marked 'mandatory' must be in place and updated as required. Those marked 'contractual' are to ensure compliance of the Service Level Agreement. Guidance and support will be provided for those marked 'Good Practice' or 'Discretionary' in the pursuit of continuous improvement to services. Any gaps identified in this

area will be supported through working together in partnership in order to improve services.

10. **Agreed Action Plan:** This is to ensure that both parties are signed up to improvement of services. Support will be provided to ensure that the plan is actioned within a reasonable, agreed time period, to be reviewed by further monitoring. The Action Plan may involve work to be undertaken by either party to the Service Level Agreement.

The monitoring template and review date will be signed by both the provider and the commissioner.

Appendix I

Section 28A Memorandum of Agreement – Annual Voucher

(This voucher may be amended to suit local arrangements. In the case of alternative providers, statutory invoicing arrangements will suffice).

Part 1 Statement of Expenditure for the Year 31st March 20...............

Scheme Ref No: ....

Title of Project: ....

Year	Capital Costs (£)	Revenue Costs (£)	Total Costs (£)
Year 1:			
Year 2:			
Year 3:			

Appendix J

A list of current NHS Foundation Trusts:

Barnsley Hospital NHS Foundation Trust

Basildon and Thurrock University Hospitals NHS Foundation Trust

Bradford Teaching Hospitals NHS Foundation Trust

Cambridge University Hospitals NHS Foundation Trust

Chesterfield Royal Hospital NHS Foundation Trust

City Hospitals Sunderland NHS Foundation Trust

Countess of Chester Hospital NHS Foundation Trust

Derby Hospitals NHS Foundation Trust

Doncaster and Bassetlaw Hospitals NHS Foundation Trust

Frimley Park Hospital NHS Foundation Trust

Gateshead Health NHS Foundation Trust

Gloucestershire Hospitals NHS Foundation Trust

Guy's and St. Thomas's NHS Foundation Trust

Harrogate and District NHS Foundation Trust

Heart of England NHS Foundation Trust

Homerton University Hospital NHS Foundation Trust

Lancashire Teaching Hospitals NHS Foundation Trust

Liverpool Women's NHS Foundation Trust

Moorfields Eye Hospital NHS Foundation Trust

Papworth Hospital NHS Foundation Trust

Peterborough and Stamford Hospitals NHS Foundation Trust

Queen Victoria Hospital NHS Foundation Trust

Royal Devon and Exeter NHS Foundation Trust

Sheffield Teaching Hospitals NHS Foundation Trust

South Tyneside NHS Foundation Trust

Stockport NHS Foundation Trust

The Rotherham NHS Foundation Trust

The Royal Bournemouth & Christchurch Hospitals NHS Foundation Trust

The Royal Marsden NHS Foundation Trust

The Royal National Hospital for Rheumatic Diseases NHS Foundation Trust

University College London Hospitals NHS Foundation Trust

University Hospital Birmingham NHS Foundation Trust

Appendix K: Working in partnership programme

Typical examples of the types of organisations involved in the working in partnership programme include:

Department of Health

NHS Modernisation Agency

Royal College of General Practitioners

The IHM

NHS Alliance

National Association of Primary Care

National Patient Safety Agency

The Association of Medical Secretaries, Practice Managers, Administrators and Receptionists (AMSPAR)

Each of the above organisations and many others are actively contributing to a wide variety of initiatives being introduced into primary care, of which practice based commissioning is just one example.

Notes

Notes